Integrative Oncology

CURRENT CLINICAL ONCOLOGY
Maurie Markman, MD, SERIES EDITOR

Integrative Oncology: Incorporating Complementary Medicine into Conventional Cancer Care, edited by LORENZO COHEN AND MAURIE MARKMAN, 2008
Prostate Cancer: Signaling Networks, Genetics and New Treatment Strategies, edited by RICHARD G. PESTELL AND MARJA T. NEVALAINEN, 2008
Intraperitoneal Cancer Therapy, edited by WILLIAM C. HELM AND ROBERT EDWARDS, 2007
Molecular Pathology of Gynecologic Cancer, edited by ANTONIO GIORDANO, ALESSANDRO BOVICELLI, AND ROBERT KURMAN, 2007
Colorectal Cancer: Evidence-Based Chemotherapy Strategies, edited by LEONARD B. SALTZ, 2007
High-Grade Gliomas: Diagnosis Treatment, edited by GENE H. BARNETT, 2006
Cancer in the Spine: Comprehensive Care, edited by ROBERT F. MCLAIN, KAI-UWE LEWANDROWSKI, MAURIE MARKMAN, RONALD M. BUKOWSKI, ROGER MACKLIS, AND EDWARD C. BENZEL, 2006
Squamous Cell Head and Neck Cancer, edited by DAVID J. ADELSTEIN, 2005
Hepatocellular Cancer: Diagnosis and Treatment, edited by BRIAN I. CARR, 2005
Biology and Management of Multiple Myeloma, edited by JAMES R. BERENSON, 2004
Cancer Immunotherapy at the Crossroads: How Tumors Evade Immunity and What Can Be Done, edited by JAMES H. FINKE AND RONALD M. BUKOWSKI, 2004
Treatment of Acute Leukemias: New Directions for Clinical Research, edited by CHING-HON PUI, 2003
Allogeneic Stem Cell Transplantation: Clinical Research and Practice, edited by MARY J. LAUGHLIN AND HILLARD M. LAZARUS, 2003
Chronic Leukemias and Lymphomas: Biology, Pathophysiology, and Clinical Management, edited by GARY J. SCHILLER, 2003
Colorectal Cancer: Multimodality Management, edited by LEONARD SALTZ, 2002
Breast Cancer: A Guide to Detection and Multidisciplinary Therapy, edited by MICHAEL H. TOROSIAN, 2002
Melanoma: Biologically Targeted Therapeutics, edited by ERNEST C. BORDEN, 2002
Cancer of the Lung: From Molecular Biology to Treatment Guidelines, edited by ALAN B. WEITBERG, 2001
Renal Cell Carcinoma: Molecular Biology, Immunology, and Clinical Management, edited by RONALD M. BUKOWSKI AND ANDREW NOVICK, 2000
Current Controversies in Bone Marrow Transplantation, edited by BRIAN J. BOLWELL, 2000
Regional Chemotherapy: Clinical Research and Practice, edited by MAURIE MARKMAN, 2000

Integrative Oncology

Incorporating Complementary Medicine into Conventional Cancer Care

Editors

Lorenzo Cohen, PhD

Director, Integrative Medicine Program
Departments of Behavioral Science and
Palliative Care and Rehabilitation Medicine
The University of Texas
M. D. Anderson Cancer Center
Houston, TX, USA

Maurie Markman, MD

Vice President for Clinical Research
Professor of Medicine
Chairman, Department of Gynecologic Medical Oncology
The University of Texas
M. D. Anderson Cancer Center
Houston, TX, USA

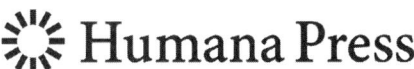

Editors

Maurie Markman
University of Texas
M. D. Anderson Cancer Center
1515 Holcombe Blvd.
Houston, TX 77030–4009, USA
mmarkman@manderson.org

Lorenzo Cohen
University of Texas
M. D. Anderson Cancer Center
1515 Holcombe Blvd.
Houston, TX 77030–4009, USA
lcohen@manderson.org

ISBN: 978-1-58829-869-0   e-ISBN: 978-1-59745-183-3

Library of Congress Control Number: 2007936725

©2008 Humana Press, a part of Springer Science+Business Media, LLC
All rights reserved. This work may not be translated or copied in whole or in part without the written permission of the publisher (Humana Press, 999 Riverview Drive, Suite 208, Totowa, NJ 07512 USA), except for brief excerpts in connection with reviews or scholarly analysis. Use in connection with any form of information storage and retrieval, electronic adaptation, computer software, or by similar or dissimilar methodology now known or hereafter developed is forbidden.
The use in this publication of trade names, trademarks, service marks, and similar terms, even if they are not identified as such, is not to be taken as an expression of opinion as to whether or not they are subject to proprietary rights.
While the advice and information in this book are believed to be true and accurate at the date of going to press, neither the authors nor the editors nor the publisher can accept any legal responsibility for any errors or omissions that may be made. The publisher makes no warranty, express or implied, with respect to the material contained herein.

Printed on acid-free paper

9 8 7 6 5 4 3 2 1

springer.com

To my wife and life partner, Alison; and our children—Alessandro, Luca, and Chiara; and to all people touched by cancer who provide the vision. (L.C.)

To my lovely wife, Tomi; and our four wonderful children, Meg, Jon, Tim, and Elisabeth. (M.M.)

Preface

Integrative oncology is a nascent field in oncology, building a rigorous evidence-based clinical medicine, research, and educational foundation. The incorporation of nonconventional treatment modalities into conventional care of people battling cancer is becoming the norm in many medical centers within the United States and around the world. As the scientific evidence mounts for the benefits of many complementary medicine treatments at helping to treat disease and manage disease- and treatment-related complications, integrative oncology will become the standard of care. International societies (Society for Integrative Oncology–www.integrativeonc.org) and journals (The Journal of the Society for Integrative Oncology) are moving the field forward and provide a forum for education and communication in integrative oncology.

Our book provides a glimpse into what is happening in the United States in the field of integrative oncology by examining five prestigious comprehensive cancer centers. Each center describes aspects of its program and provides the reader with valuable information about starting integrative oncology at their center. Critical areas in integrative oncology are also covered, including potential harm, legal issues, and how to communicate with patients.

We believe this book provides a valuable resource for starting integrative oncology at other medical centers, clinics, and private practices around the world. The appropriate and safe integration of complementary medicine within conventional cancer care will help to improve the lives of the millions of people affected by cancer worldwide.

Lorenzo Cohen
Maurie Markman

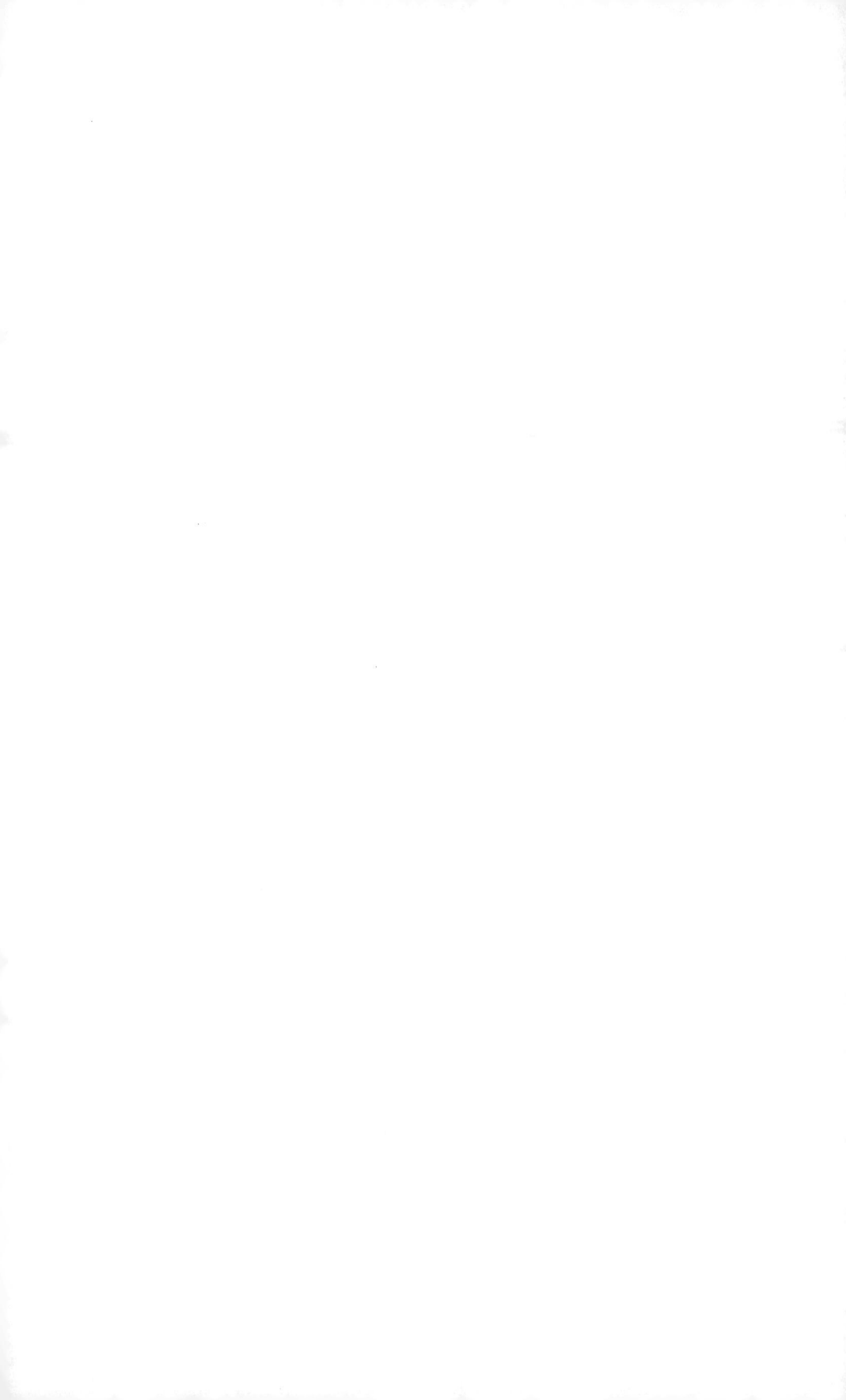

Contents

Integrative Oncology Overview

1 **Introduction** 3
   Lorenzo Cohen and Maurie Markman

2 **A Word of Caution:** *Risk of Harm Associated with Alternative Complementary/Integrative Approaches in Cancer Management and the Critical Need for Quality Research to Understand and Decrease that Risk* 9
   Maurie Markman

3 **Using Legal and Ethical Principles to Guide Clinical Decision Making in Complementary/Integrative Cancer Medicine** 15
   Michael H. Cohen

4 **Communicating with Patients about the Use of Complementary and Integrative Medicine in Cancer Care** 33
   Moshe Frenkel and Eran Ben-Arye

Integrative Oncology Programs at National Cancer Institute Comprehensive Cancer Centers

5 **The Integrative Medicine Program at The University of Texas M. D. Anderson Cancer Center** 49
   Lorenzo Cohen, Laura Baynham-Fletcher, and Catherine Kirkwood

6 **The Integrative Medicine Service at Memorial Sloan-Kettering Cancer Center** 67
   Barrie Cassileth and Jyothirmai Gubili

7 **Integrative Oncology—Leonard P. Zakim Center:** *The Dana-Farber Cancer Institute Experience* 79
   David S. Rosenthal, Anne Doherty-Gilman, Cynthia Medeiros, Susan DeCristofaro, and Elizabeth Dean-Clower

8 **The Johns Hopkins Complementary and Integrative Medicine Service** 105
   Kathleen Menten, Sanghoon Lee, and Adrian S. Dobs

9 **Integrative Oncology at Mayo Clinic:** *Research Informing Practice* 123
   Debra L. Barton, Brent A. Bauer and Charles L. Loprinzi

The Research

10 **Mind–Body Research in Cancer** 139
    Kavita D. Chandwani, Alejandro Chaoul-Reich, Kelly A. Biegler, and Lorenzo Cohen

11 **Herbs and Other Botanicals: Interactions with Pharmaceuticals** 161
    Jyothirmai Gubili, Simon Yeung, and Barrie Cassileth

12 **Acupuncture in Cancer Care at Dana-Farber Cancer Institute:** *An Integrative Medical Practice* 181
    Weidong Lu, Elizabeth Dean-Clower, Anne Doherty-Gilman and David S. Rosenthal

13 **Acupuncture for the Side Effects of Cancer Treatments** 201
    Sanghoon Lee, Kathleen Menten, and Adrian S. Dobs

Index 213

Contributors

Brent A. Bauer, MD, FACP
Director Complementary and
 Integrative Medicine Program
Mayo Clinic
Rochester, MN, USA

Laura Baynham-Fletcher, MD, FACP
Department of Palliative Care and
 Rehabilitation Medicine
The University of Texas
M. D. Anderson Cancer Center
Houston, TX, USA

Eran Ben-Arye, MD
The Complementary and
 Traditional Medicine Unit
Department of Family Medicine
The Bruce Rappaport Faculty
 of Medicine
The Technion, Israel Institute
 of Technology
Clalit Health Services
Haifa and Western Galilee District
Haifa, Israel

Debra L. Barton RN, PhD
Cancer Center
Mayo Clinic
Rochester, MN, USA

Kelly A. Biegler, PhD
Integrative Medicine Program
The University of Texas
M. D. Anderson Cancer Center
Houston, TX, USA

Barrie Cassileth, MS, PhD
Integrative Medicine Service
Memorial Sloan-Kettering Cancer
 Center, New York, NY, USA

Kavita D. Chandwani, MD, MPH
Department of Behavioral Science
The University of Texas
M. D. Anderson Cancer Center
Houston, TX, USA

Alejandro Chaoul-Reich, PhD
Department of Palliative Care
 and Rehabilitation Medicine
The University of Texas
M. D. Anderson Cancer Center
Houston, TX, USA

Lorenzo Cohen, PhD
Director, Integrative Medicine Program
Departments of Behavioral Science and
Palliative Care and Rehabilitation
 Medicine
The University of Texas
M. D. Anderson Cancer Center
Houston, TX, USA

Michael H. Cohen, JD, MBA, MFA
Principal Law Offices of
 Michael H. Cohen
Cambridge, MA, USA

Elizabeth Dean-Clower, MD, MPH
Leonard P. Zakim Center
  for Integrative Therapies
Dana-Farber Cancer Institute
Boston, MA, USA

Susan DeCristofaro, RN, MS, OCN
Leonard P. Zakim Center
  for Integrative Therapies
Dana-Farber Cancer Institute
Boston, MA, USA

Adrian S. Dobs, MD, MHS
Professor of Medicine and Oncology
Division of Endocrinology and
  Metabolism
Johns Hopkins University School
  of Medicine
Baltimore, MD, USA

Anne Doherty-Gilman, MPH
Program Manager Leonard P. Zakim
  Center for Integrative Therapies
Dana-Farber
Cancer Institute
Boston, MA, USA

Moshe Frenkel, MD
Medical Director
Integrative Medicine Program
The University of Texas
M. D. Anderson Cancer Center
Houston, TX, USA

Jyothirmai Gubili, MS
Integrative Medicine Service
Memorial Sloan-Kettering Cancer
  Center
New York, NY, USA

Catherine Kirkwood, MS
Department of Palliative Care and
  Rehabilitation Medicine
The University of Texas
M. D. Anderson Cancer Center
Houston, TX, USA

Sanghoon Lee, KMD, PhD, LAc
Research Fellow, The Johns Hopkins
Center for Complementary and
  Alternative Medicine
Division of Endocrinology and
  Metabolism Oncology Center
Department of Acupuncture
  and Moxibustion
College of Korean Medicine
Kyung Hee University
Seoul, Korea

Charles L. Loprinzi, MD
Department of Oncology
Mayo Clinic
Rochester, MN, USA

Weidong Lu, M.B., MPH, Lic.Ac.
Leonard P. Zakim Center for Integrative
  Therapies
Dana-Farber Cancer Institute
Research Fellow
Harvard Medical School
Boston, MA, USA
Professor of Chinese Medicine
The New England School
  of Acupuncture
Newton, MA, USA

Maurie Markman, MD
Vice President for Clinical Research
Professor of Medicine
Chairman, Department of Gynecologic
  Medical Oncology
The University of Texas
M. D. Anderson Cancer Center
Houston, TX, USA

Cynthia Medeiros, MSW, LICSW
Director
Patient Care Service Administration
Dana-Farber Cancer Institute
Boston, MA, USA

Kathleen Menten, RN, MSN, LAc
Program Coordinator, Complementary
  and Integrative Medicine Service
  in Oncology
Johns Hopkins University School
  of Medicine,
Baltimore, MD, USA

David S. Rosenthal, MD
Director, Harvard University
  Health Service
Co-Director, Zakim Center
  for Integrative Therapies

Dana-Farber Cancer Institute
Professor of Medicine
Harvard Medical School
Henry K. Oliver Professor of Hygiene
  Harvard University
Cambridge, MA, USA

Simon Yeung, MBA, PharmD, LAC
Integrative Medicine Service
Memorial Sloan-Kettering Cancer
  Center
New York, NY, USA

Integrative Oncology Overview

Chapter 1
Introduction

Lorenzo Cohen and Maurie Markman

Abstract The use of complementary and alternative medicine (CAM) and the practice of integrative medicine has been steadily growing for the past 20 years. The growth has been partially driven by the population's utilization of CAM and also by the increase in scientific evidence supporting the use of different treatments. Many medical centers within the United States have formalized integrative medicine programs to help guide patients in the use of CAM and to provide CAM services. This book outlines integrative medicine programs at five leading National Cancer Institute Comprehensive Cancer Centers. The focus is on how these centers started their programs, what they are currently doing, and recommendations for starting integrative medicine clinics. Four of the centers also describe in more detail specifics for one aspect of their research program. This allows the reader to see one aspect of the research that is being done in more detail. Some chapters also focus on more general topics such as the potential harm from CAM, legal issues surrounding CAM, and how to communicate with patients about CAM. This book is for people wanting to start integrative medicine programs and to improve the care for people with cancer across the nation and the world.

Keywords: Oncology · integrative medicine · complementary medicine · cancer centers.

Complementary and alternative medicine (CAM) has been defined by the National Center for Complementary and Alternative Medicine (NCCAM) and major U.S. surveys as "... diverse medical and healthcare systems, practices, and products that are not presently considered to be part of conventional medicine" [1]. Some CAM approaches are completely unconventional while others are borderline conventional or actually conventional but not in the setting in which they are being used. The terminology used to describe these CAM approaches can be confusing.

L. Cohen
Director, Integrative Medicine Program, M. D. Anderson Cancer Center, 1515 Holcombe Blvd., Unit # 145, Houston TX 77030
e-mail: lcohen@mdanderson.org

The terms "complementary" and "alternative" are often used interchangeably, but they describe two different approaches. Alternative medicine is defined as a treatment modality used in place of conventional medicine. By definition, alternative treatments are not integrated as part of conventional medicine. Complementary medicine, however, makes use of non-conventional treatment modalities, some of which have known efficacy, in combination with conventional treatment. Both alternative and complementary medicine focus on treatment modalities. Integrative medicine, on the other hand, is not about specific non-conventional treatment modalities, but is an approach to treating patients. It strives to integrate the best of complementary and conventional modalities using a multidisciplinary approach through integrative services. The Consortium of Academic Health Centers for Integrative Medicine has recently defined integrative medicine as the practice of medicine that reaffirms the importance of the relationship between practitioner and patient, focuses on the whole person, is informed by evidence, and makes use of all appropriate therapeutic approaches, providers, and disciplines to achieve optimal health and healing [2].

Complementary therapies typically used include mind-body approaches such as meditation, guided imagery, music, art, other expressive arts, and other behavioral techniques; energy-based therapies that seek to affect proposed bio-energy fields, whose existence is not yet experimentally proven, that surround and penetrate the human body. These can be individual therapies done through self-practice (e.g. Yoga, Tai Chi, or internal Qigong), manipulation of electromagnetic waves through the use of magnets, or through the use of the energy of individual practitioners (e.g., external Qigong, Reiki, Healing Touch); body-manipulative systems such as chiropractic and massage; alternative medical systems such as traditional Chinese medicine, homeopathy, and Ayurveda (Indian-based medicine); and biologically based approaches such as nutrition, herbal/plant, animal/mineral, or other products.

CAM is used by an estimated 35–36% of U.S. adults according to surveys in 1997 and 2002 [3,4], 62% if prayer is included [3]. CAM use is particularly prevalent among patients with cancer. For patients with cancer being treated in comprehensive cancer centers in the United States, the rate of CAM use varies from 48 to 88% [5–7]. People who use complementary therapies are often seeking a more holistic and noninvasive approach to preventing and managing disease. They use CAM to maintain wellness, improve quality of life, assist in managing disease- and treatment-related side effects, boost the immune system, increase hope, and gain a sense of control [8,9].

Some types of complementary treatments have a place in the treatment of cancer and cancer-related side effects, and much research is currently being done in this area. Acupuncture, for example, may reduce chemotherapy-induced nausea and post-operative vomiting [10,11], St. John's wort is useful in helping to manage mild to moderate depression [12], and many mind-body programs can buffer the symptoms caused by conventional cancer treatments [13]. However, some forms of CAM are associated with risks, especially in patients with cancer, and thus it is important that oncologists be aware of complementary therapies their patients are using.

Even though people with cancer typically use complementary medicines along with their conventional treatment, anywhere from 38 to 60% of patients with cancer do so without informing any member of their health care team [3, 7]. This lack of discussion is of grave concern, especially for ingestible substances (herbs, supplements, vitamins, special diets, medicinal teas, etc.). There are a variety of reasons why open communication about complementary treatments is not taking place in the medical clinics. The most common reason patients give is that it just never came up in the discussion, that is, no one asked them, and they did not think it was important. Patients may fear that the topic will be received with indifference or dismissed without discussion, and health care professionals may fear not knowing how to respond to questions or fear initiating a time-consuming discussion [6, 7].

Interest and support for CAM research has steadily grown over the past 16 years. The Office of Alternative Medicine was established at the National Institutes of Health back in 1991 with a budget of $2 million. The purpose of the Office was to investigate and evaluate promising unconventional medical practices [14]. In 1998, the office was raised to the level of center and named the National Center for Complementary and Alternative Medicine. The current mission of NCCAM is:

> The National Center for Complementary and Alternative Medicine (NCCAM) is dedicated to exploring complementary and alternative healing practices in the context of rigorous science; training complementary and alternative medicine researchers; and disseminating authoritative information to the public and professionals. To fulfill its mission, the NCCAM supports a broad-based portfolio of research, research training, and educational grants and contracts, as well as various outreach mechanisms to disseminate information.

NCCAM has a broad research portfolio that focuses in all CAM domains:

> NCCAM's primary responsibility is the conduct and support of basic and clinical research studies, using well-established tools of rigorous scientific design, conduct and oversight. These studies involve investigator-initiated projects as well as NCCAM-solicited applications. Examples include large, multi-center clinical trials; CAM Specialty Centers of Research; studies of therapies from whole medical systems (e.g., Ayurvedic medicine and traditional Chinese medicine); and studies in the four domains of CAM: manipulative and body-based therapies, biologically based practices, mind-body medicine, and energy medicine. The Center carries out these activities independently and in collaboration with other NIH Institutes and Centers, other government agencies, domestic and international research institutions, and industry.

In 1998, NCCAM had an annual budget of $40.5 million and it has increased to a request of $119.1 for fiscal year 2007. Importantly, many other Institutes and Offices are investing in CAM research, with an estimated total funding, including NCCAM, of over $300 million. Although this is just a fraction of the total NIH budget, tremendous progress is being made in determining the efficacy or lack of efficacy of certain treatments (i.e., therapeutic methods) and understanding some of the mechanisms of action (e.g., acupuncture) [14].

The institute with the most interest and investment in CAM research is by far the National Cancer Institute (NCI). In 1998, the NCI established The Office of Cancer Complementary and Alternative Medicine (OCCAM) to "coordinate and enhance the activities of the NCI with regard to complementary and alternative medicine (CAM)." The OCCAM's goal is to:

> Increase the amount of high-quality cancer research and information about the use of complementary and alternative modalities by:
>
> Promoting and supporting research of CAM disciplines and modalities as they relate to the prevention, diagnosis, and treatment of cancer, cancer-related symptoms and side effects of conventional treatment.
>
> Coordinating NCI's CAM research and information activities.
>
> Coordinating NCI's collaboration with other governmental and non-governmental organizations on CAM cancer issues.
>
> Providing an interface with health practitioners and researchers regarding CAM cancer issues.

The NCI portfolio of extramural and intramural research funding in CAM for cancer has expanded dramatically since 1998 when the annual expenditures were under $30 million to approximately $124 million for fiscal year 2006. The NCI supports a broad range of research including R03's, R13's, R21's, R01's, U19's, and U01's within all the CAM categories. The OCCAM also has a less conventional venue for examining CAM approaches and that is what is called the NCI Best Case Series Program. Since 1991, the NCI has utilized this program to evaluate data from CAM practitioners with the same rigorous scientific methods employed in evaluating treatment responses with conventional medicine [15, 16]. This program provides an independent review of medical records and medical imaging from patients treated with unconventional cancer therapies. Staff from the OCCAM work with CAM practitioners to identify appropriate, well-documented cases. The primary goal of the program is to obtain and review sufficient information to determine if NCI-initiated research on a specific intervention is warranted [17]. The support for research in integrative oncology is especially important as the majority of people diagnosed with cancer, as noted above, use some form of CAM.

Many medical centers within the United States have formalized integrative medicine programs to help guide patients in the use of CAM and to provide CAM services. Starting an integrative medicine clinic, whether it is small and offers only a few services or it is a large center offering many services, conducting research, and supporting educational programming, is a daunting task. This book outlines integrative medicine programs at five leading National Cancer Institute Comprehensive Cancer Centers (The University of Texas M. D. Anderson Cancer Center, Memorial Sloan Kettering Cancer Center, Dana Farber Cancer Institute, The Johns Hopkins Kimmel Oncology Cancer Center, and the Mayo Clinic). The focus is on how these centers started their programs, what they are currently doing, and recommendations for starting integrative medicine clinics. Four of the centers also describe in more detail specifics for one aspect of their research program (M. D. Anderson Cancer Center Kimmel Oncology Cancer Center: Mind-body research; Memorial Sloan Kettering Cancer Center: Botanical research; Dana Farber Cancer Institute: Chinese acupuncture research; and The Johns Hopkins: Korean acupuncture). This allows the reader to see one aspect of the research that is being done in more detail. Important chapters also focus on more general topics such as the potential harm from CAM, legal issues surround CAM, and how to communicate with patients about CAM. We hope this book is helpful to people wanting to start integrative medicine programs and to improve the care for people with cancer across the nation and the world.

References

1. NCCAM. What is complementary and alternative medicine? http://nccam.nih.gov/health/whatiscam/. Accessed April 2007.
2. CAHCIM. http://www.imconsortium.org/cahcim/about/home.html. Accessed April 2007.
3. Barnes P, Powell-Griner E, McFann K, Nathin R. CDC Advance Data Report #343: Complementary and Alternative Medicine Use Among Adults: United States, 2002. May 27, 2004 Report No.: 343.
4. Tindle HA, Davis RB, Phillips RS, Eisenberg DM. Trends in use of complementary and alternative medicine by US adults: 1997–2002. Altern Ther Health Med 2005 Jan–Feb;11(1):42–9.
5. Dy GK, Bekele L, Hanson LJ, Furth A, Mandrekar S, Sloan JA, et al. Complementary and alternative medicine use by patients enrolled onto phase I clinical trials. J Clin Oncol 2004 Dec 1;22(23):4810–5.
6. Navo MA, Phan J, Vaughan C, Palmer JL, Michaud L, Jones KL, et al. An assessment of the utilization of complementary and alternative medication in women with gynecologic or breast malignancies. J Clin Oncol 2004;22(4):671–7.
7. Richardson MA, Sanders T, Palmer JL, Greisinger A, Singletary SE. Complementary/alternative medicine use in a comprehensive cancer center and the implications for oncology. J Clin Oncol 2000;18(13):2505–14.
8. Eisenberg DM, Kessler RC, Van Rompay MI, Kaptchuk TJ, Wilkey SA, Appel S, et al. Perceptions about complementary therapies relative to conventional therapies among adults who use both: results from a national survey. Ann Intern Med 2001 Sep 4;135(5):344–51.
9. Richardson MA, Masse LC, Nanny K, Sanders C. Discrepant views of oncologists and cancer patients on complementary/alternative medicine. Support Care Cancer 2004 Nov;12(11):797–804.
10. Ezzo J, Vickers A, Richardson MA, Allen C, Dibble SL, Issell B, et al. Acupuncture-point stimulation for chemotherapy-induced nausea and vomiting. J Clin Oncol 2005 Oct 1;23(28):7188–98.
11. Lee A, Done ML. The use of nonpharmacologic techniques to prevent postoperative nausea and vomiting: a meta-analysis. Anesth Analg 1999 Jun;88(6):1362–9.
12. Linde K, Mulrow CD, Berner M, Egger M. St John's wort for depression. Cochrane Database Syst Rev 2005(2):CD000448.
13. Astin JA, Shapiro SL, Eisenberg DM, Forys KL. Mind-body medicine: state of the science, implications for practice. J Am Board Fam Pract 2003 Mar–Apr;16(2):131–47.
14. NCCAM. http://nccam.nih.gov/. Accessed April 2007.
15. Hawkins MJ, Friedman MA. National Cancer Institute's evaluation of unconventional cancer treatments. J Natl Cancer Inst 1992;84(22):1699–702.
16. Lee CO. Translational research in cancer complementary and alternative medicine: the National Cancer Institute's Best Case Series Program. Clin J Oncol Nurs 2004;8(2):212–4.
17. NCI-OCCAM. http://www.cancer.gov/cam/. Accessed April 2007.

Chapter 2
A Word of Caution

Risk of Harm Associated with Alternative Complementary/Integrative Approaches in Cancer Management and the Critical Need for Quality Research to Understand and Decrease that Risk

Maurie Markman

Contents

2.1 Risk of "Harm" Associated with "Non-conventional" Approaches to Cancer Management 10
2.2 Direct Harmful Effects of Non-traditional Strategies 11
2.3 Conclusion 12
References 12

Abstract Despite the perception of some that so-called natural pharmaceutical approaches to cancer disease management are completely safe, rather extensive data in the peer-reviewed medical literature has revealed the potential toxicities associated with a number of such strategies. It will be important for the oncology research community to thoroughly evaluate all claims of safety for any medication used in the cancer patient population. Concerns include both the side effects of the drugs/herbs themselves and the potential for interactions with established anti-cancer agents.

Keywords: Cancer chemotherapy · toxicity of pharmaceutical agents · management of advanced cancer · herbal medications.

Interest by cancer patients in complementary and alternative medicine (CAM) non-conventional strategies in the management of their illness are well recognized [1–3]. While patients have different reasons for employing a remarkably diverse group of such approaches, one recurring theme in essentially all reports of these activities is the desire of patients to do all in their power to favorably influence their

---

M. Markman
VP, Clinical Research, M. D. Anderson Cancer Center, 1515 Holcombe Blvd., Unit # 121, Houston, TX 77030
e-mail: mmarkman@mdanderson.org

own outcome, whether this is an improvement in survival or a reduction in side effects of treatment [4, 5].

As the impressive content of this book clearly demonstrates, the academic medical community has taken notice of this important patient-centered paradigm and has initiated clinical programs and highly relevant research efforts designed to ultimately assist patients in their exploration of beneficial strategies.

2.1 Risk of "Harm" Associated with "Non-conventional" Approaches to Cancer Management

One legitimate concern regarding the use of CAM is the potential for *harm*. Considered broadly, harm in the context of the current discussion can take several forms (Table 2.1).

For example, a patient may feel intense disappointment when a desired outcome did not occur (e.g., use of a "herbal medication" did not "cure" what is recognized to be an incurable cancer) [6].

Another type of harm can result, more serious in its impact on a measurable outcome, if a patient elects to pursue a non-conventional unproven strategy claimed to be "natural and non-toxic" rather than a well-established highly effective conventional treatment approach associated with recognized unpleasant, but rarely life-threatening, acute or chronic side effects (e.g., cisplatin-based combination chemotherapy as therapy for a metastatic germ cell tumor) [7, 8]. In this specific

Table 2.1 Potential "Harms" Associated with Alternative/Complementary/Integrative Approaches to Cancer Management

1. Impact of disappointment associated with the realization that the profoundly unrealistic expectations for a favorable outcome will not occur (e.g., "cure" of rapidly progressive chemotherapy-resistant widely metastatic cancer)
2. Personal decision to employ "alternative" management strategy rather than highly effective *conventional medical treatment* resulting in severe consequences (e.g., death from failure to administer curative chemotherapy for germ cell tumors, leukemia, lymphomas; profound suffering related to attempt of patient to "eliminate natural substances from body" including narcotic analgesia given for severe cancer-related pain)
3. Side effects associated with unregulated and unsafe delivery of non-conventional interventions [e.g., serious intestinal infections associated with "pursing enemas" [10]]
4. Direct toxic effects on normal organ function [e.g., hydrazine sulfate leading to hepatic failure [20]; laetrile-associated cyanide toxicity [21, 22]]
5. Increase in the toxicity of conventional cancer treatment
6. Toxicity of non-conventional approach mistakenly ascribed to effects of cancer treatment [e.g., emesis secondary to laetrile [21, 22]]
7. Interference with favorable biological activity of conventional treatment [e.g., St. John's wort increasing hepatic metabolism of irinotecan and docetaxel [15, 18]]
8. Biological effect of a non-conventional product incorrectly assumed to be the result of progressive cancer [e.g., "over-the-counter" vitamin D preparations leading to hypercalcemia believed to be caused by metastatic disease in bone [23]]

and hopefully uncommon situation, the decision by the patient to employ the "alternative" strategy may tragically result in avoidable death.

Non-conventional management strategies may also be delivered in settings where the "standard" regulatory environment, designed to insure safety of medical interventions, does not apply. Absence of such safeguards can result in potentially serious consequences. For example, a preparation claimed to "augment the immune system" of cancer patients and administered at an unregulated "off-shore clinic" was shown to contain hepatitis virus [9]. In another completely unregulated unsanitary "clinic" environment, the use of enemas, claimed to "purge the body of cancer sustaining toxins," has been documented to lead to severe, and even fatal, intestinal infections [10].

A far more subtle, but no less serious "harm," of non-conventional therapy relates to the claim of some alternative care providers that their prescribed "natural cure" can only be effective if all *"unnatural substances"* are eliminated from the body. Such "unnatural substances" include narcotic analgesia employed by patients to control cancer-related pain or chemotherapy to help control the cancer. Thus, these providers have a ready-made excuse for why their "treatment" did not *"cure the cancer"* ("I told the patient this natural therapy would not be effective if unnatural substances remained in the body"). However, of far greater concern is the fact a desperate patient may endure profound suffering and intense pain in a futile attempt to discontinue the only treatment making their remaining days bearable.

2.2 Direct Harmful Effects of Non-traditional Strategies

Both conventional and non-conventional management strategies have the potential to cause harm to a patient either by directly interfering with normal organ function or by potentiating the risks of toxicity or interfering with the beneficial effects of another intervention [11–13].

One of the most problematic aspects of CAM strategies, that innovative research being conducted at a number of academic medical programs is attempting to correct, is the absence of data confirming the safety of these agents in specific clinical settings [14].

For example, while St. John's wort is widely employed as a "safe" treatment for depression, it is now well established the drug can enhance the hepatic metabolism of several important pharmaceutical agents, including cyclosporine, irinotecan, imatinib mesylate and docetaxel [15–18]. The medical literature has documented the profoundly serious problem of the loss of a number of life-sustaining transplanted organs (heart, kidney) as a result of inadequate cyclosporine blood levels in individuals who elected to take St. John's wort [19].

In the case of the use of anti-cancer drugs in individuals who are also self-administering St. John's wort, there is legitimate concern that the reduced concentrations of the anti-neoplastic agents may substantially decrease their effectiveness.

For how many other conventional anti-cancer agents is their metabolism, and clearance, influenced by the simultaneous use of St. John's wort? Furthermore are there other commonly employed CAM approaches that can affect the biological activity or safety of anti-neoplastic treatment? These questions are certainly highly worthy of investigation by the academic oncology community.

There is also the concern about quality of products as the Food and Drug Administration does not regulate most products that are classified as CAM supplements, herbs and other ingestible substances. There is the possibility that during the manufacturing of the product, dangerous contaminants can be included. If the manufacturing is not done using good manufacturing practices, then there could also be issues of having the appropriate doses of the active ingredient (either getting too much or too little).

2.3 Conclusion

It is important to clearly state the intent of this chapter has not been to claim, or even suggest, that the group of personal interventions employed in the cancer patient population and loosely classified together as "complementary/integrative" are particularly dangerous or unusually toxic.

Rather, the point to be made is that *all interventions* in this clinical setting, whether conventional or non-conventional, have the potential to produce harm, both minor (e.g., disappointment the hoped for outcome did not occur) and major (e.g., chemotherapy-associated neutropenic sepsis or neuropathy; avoidable death due to the decision to employ an untested and unproven "alternative" strategy).

In addition, in often striking contrast to the situation of conventional medical strategies, there is frequently a complete absence of data regarding the potential for such harm associated with the use of non-conventional approaches. Thus, it is the lack of information regarding safety, rather than documented serious toxic effects that are most concerning about the unregulated and unsupervised use of this group of interventions.

As a result, the efforts of the academic medical community to study a variety of CAM strategies are a critically important, and profoundly necessary, development.

References

1. Ernst E, Cassileth BR. The prevalence of complementary/alternative medicine in cancer: a systematic review. Cancer 1998; 83:777–782.
2. Lafferty WE, Bellas A, Corage BA, et al. The use of complementary and alternative medical providers by insured cancer patients in Washington state. Cancer 2004; 100:1522–1530.
3. Dy GK, Bekele L, Hanson LJ, et al. Complementary and alternative medicine use by patients enrolled onto phase I clinical trials. J Clin Oncol 2004; 22:4810–4815.
4. Cassileth BR, Lusk EJ, Strouse TB, et al. Contemporary unorthodox treatments in cancer medicine. A study of patients, treatments, and practitioners. Ann Intern Med 1984; 101: 105–112.
5. Sollner W, Maislinger S, Devries A, et al. Use of complementary and alternative medicine by cancer patients is not associated with perceived distress or poor compliance with standard treatment but with active coping behavior: a survey. Cancer 2000; 89:873–880.

6. Schofield P, Ball D, Smith JG, et al. Optimism and survival in lung carcinoma patients. Cancer 2004; 100:1276–1282.
7. Coppes MJ, Anderson RA, Egeler RM, et al. Alternative therapies for the treatment of childhood cancer. N Engl J Med 1998; 339:846–847.
8. Ernst E. Intangible risks of complementary and alternative medicine. J Clin Oncol 2001; 19:2365–2366.
9. Green S. Immunoaugmentative therapy. An unproven cancer treatment. JAMA 1993; 270:1719–1723.
10. Markman M. Medical complications of "alternative" cancer therapy. N Engl J Med 1985; 312:1640–1641 (letter).
11. Sparreboom A, Cox MC, Acharya MR, et al. Herbal remedies in the United States: potential adverse interactions with anticancer agents. J Clin Oncol 2004; 22:2489–2503.
12. Morris CA, Avorn J. Internet marketing of herbal products. JAMA 2003; 290:1505–1509.
13. Werneke U, Earl J, Seydel C, et al. Potential health risks of complementary alternative medicines in cancer patients. Br J Cancer 2004; 90:408–413.
14. Marwick C. Complementary, alternative therapies should face rigorous testing, IOM concludes. J Natl Cancer Inst 2005; 97:255–256.
15. Komoroski BJ, Parise RA, Egorin MJ, et al. Effect of the St. John's wort constituent hyperforin on docetaxel metabolism by human hepatocyte cultures. Clin Cancer Res 2005;11:6972–6979.
16. Smith P, Bullock JM, Booker BM, et al. The influence of St. John's wort on the pharmacokinetics and protein binding of imatinib mesylate. Pharmacotherapy 2004; 24:1508–1514.
17. Frye RF, Fitzgerald SM, Lagattuta TF, et al. Effect of St John's wort on imatinib mesylate pharmacokinetics. Clin Pharmacol Ther 2004; 76:323–329.
18. Mathijssen RH, Verweij J, de Bruijn P, et al. Effects of St. John's wort on irinotecan metabolism. J Natl Cancer Inst 2002; 94:1247–1249.
19. Ruschitzka F, Meier PJ, Turina M, et al. Acute heart transplant rejection due to Saint John's wort. Lancet 2000; 355:548–549.
20. Hainer MI, Tsai N, Komura ST, et al. Fatal hepatorenal failure associated with hydrazine sulfate. Ann Intern Med 2000; 133:877–880.
21. Moertel CG, Ames MM, Kovach JS, et al. A pharmacologic and toxicological study of amygdalin. JAMA 1981; 245:591–594.
22. Dorr RT, Paxinos J. The current status of laetrile. Ann Intern Med 1978; 89:389–397.
23. Koutkia P, Chen TC, Holick MF. Vitamin D intoxication associated with an over-the-counter supplement. N Engl J Med 2001; 345:66–67.

Chapter 3
Using Legal and Ethical Principles to Guide Clinical Decision Making in Complementary/Integrative Cancer Medicine

Michael H. Cohen

Contents

3.1	Introduction	15
3.2	Major Applicable Legal Rules	16
3.3	Malpractice Issues in Greater Detail	20
3.4	Some Ways to Help Manage Liability Risks	26
3.5	The Federation of State Medical Board Guidelines for Integrative Medicine	27
3.6	A Broader Ethical Analysis	28
3.7	Conclusion	30
References		31

Abstract The integration of complementary and alternative medical (CAM) therapies into cancer medicine raises legal issues for clinicians who may be initiating delivery of CAM therapies, referring patients to CAM providers, or simply responding to patient requests concerning specific CAM modalities. This chapter addresses some of the key legal issues and liability risk management strategies legal issues and liability risk management strategies in order to help guide oncologists regarding a clinically and legally defensible approach to inclusion of CAM therapies in cancer medicine.

Keywords: Liability · medical malpractice · informed consent · complementary and alternative medicine · cancer medicine.

3.1 Introduction

Use of complementary and alternative medical (CAM) therapies (such as acupuncture and traditional oriental medicine, chiropractic, herbal medicine, massage therapy, and "mind-body" therapies such as hypnotherapy and guided imagery) in

---

M. Cohen
Principal, Law Offices of Michael H. Cohen, 770, Massachusetts Avenue, Suite 391108, Cambridge, MA 02139

cancer medicine raises legal issues for clinicians who may be initiating delivery of CAM therapies, referring patients to CAM providers, or simply responding to patient requests concerning specific CAM modalities. Clinical integration of CAM therapies into conventional care generally also raises legal and issues for institutions, which must negotiate between the competing demands of their various constituencies to satisfy administrative, legal, and patient care concerns [1–3].

Thorough understanding of legal and ethical issues is important to clinical decision making involving integration of CAM therapies, while inadequate understanding can jeopardize patient care [4]. Specifically, ignorance of legal and ethical issues on one hand and undue fear of liability concerns or misunderstanding of ethical questions on the other can distort patient care by resulting in either dangerous inclusion of risky CAM therapies on one side or under-inclusion of potentially helpful CAM therapies on the other. Put another way, the combination of ignorance and fear regarding legal issues creates a "double-edged sword: beneficial CAM therapies are under-utilized in the realms of prevention and supportive care; dangerous interactions can exist between some CAM and conventional treatments; and delays in beginning conventional treatment can result in cancer dissemination and death" [5]. This chapter addresses some of the key legal issues and liability risk management strategies in order to help guide oncologists regarding a clinically and legally defensible approach to inclusion of CAM therapies in cancer medicine.

3.2 Major Applicable Legal Rules

One definition of "integrative oncology" describes this emerging field as "a comprehensive, evidence-based approach to cancer care that addresses all participants at all levels of their being and experience" [5]. This definition adapts current notions of "integrative medicine"—the judicious integration of CAM and conventional therapies in the best interest of the patient—to oncology, with emphasis on aspects of patient care including attention to "body, mind, soul and spirit within the self, and within the specific culture and the natural world" [5]. According to this perspective, one of the reasons for the "push and pull" driving patients (and many clinicians and institutions) to understand the boundaries of CAM therapies in cancer medicine has to do with renewed emphasis on the possible contribution of self-care, the desire to increase patient control, and possible improved outcomes [5].

Such currents within medicine and the medical marketplace will surely also affect the evolution of law. However, current law does not define "integrative medicine," and historically, statutes and judicial opinions in the United States did not define the terms "alternative" or "complementary" medicine. State statutes do define the practice of "medicine," as well as other professional healing arts (where licensed), such as chiropractic, acupuncture and traditional oriental medicine, and massage therapy.

But more generally, it is useful to look at the cross-section of laws governing the healing arts that relate to the CAM professions, or that relate to the matter of conventional practitioners (such as licensed medical doctors) including CAM therapies in discussions with patients. From this vantage, some basic principles of health law apply whether a therapy is labeled "conventional" or "CAM" [6]. Seven critical principles that can be applied across therapies and professions involve (1) licensure; (2) scope of practice; (3) malpractice liability; (4) professional discipline; (5) access to treatments; (6) third-party reimbursement; and (7) healthcare fraud [6].

These areas are broadly described with case examples elsewhere [6], though it is worth briefly summarizing some of the major legal rules that would apply whether discussing integrative pediatrics, oncology, cardiology, or any other specialty, and identifying how these rules might especially apply to cancer medicine and integration of CAM therapies in cancer medicine.

3.2.1 Licensure and Credentialing

Licensure refers to the requirement in most states that healthcare providers maintain a current state license to practice their professional healing art. Historically, medical licensing statutes made the unlicensed practice of "medicine" a crime and defined the practice of "medicine" broadly in terms of "diagnosis" and "treatment" of "any human disease" or "condition" [6]. This put non-licensed practitioners of the healing arts at risk of prosecution for unlawful medical practice. Over time, chiropractors, massage therapists, naturopathic physicians, acupuncturists, and other CAM providers gained licensure on a state-by-state basis [6].

Today, while a few states have enacted statutes authorizing non-licensed, CAM providers to practice with certain restrictions [7], in most states, licensure serves as the first hurdle to professional practice. The existence of licensure for the various CAM providers varies by state; chiropractors, for example, are licensed in every state, whereas massage therapists and acupuncturists are licensed in well over half the states, and naturopathic physicians in at least a dozen states [8].

Licensing for CAM providers is not uniform across states, perhaps frustrating practitioners used to more standardized educational and licensure requirements for conventional healthcare providers such as the various board-certified medical specialists [8]. Furthermore, CAM practitioners often have relatively modest training in medical sciences, or may focus more on subjects such as anatomy and physiology (e.g., for massage therapists) and less on subjects such as biochemistry [8]. Some practitioners may operate within spheres of knowledge foreign to biomedicine—for example, acupuncture meridian theory; many may lack familiarity with tools of medical research including principles of evidence-based medicine and methods for analyzing research data reported in the medical literature. Furthermore, licensure is meant to represent a given level of competence, though it provides no guarantee of quality assurance [6]. Some states will grant title licensure but allow practitioners at a lower threshold of training to practice so long as they do not use the designated title (e.g., providers in some states might be allowed to counsel patients so long as they do not call themselves "psychologists") [6].

In view of these issues concerning licensure, credentialing refers to the verification of practitioner credentials to ensure competence, whether the practitioner is considered a conventional healthcare provider delivering a CAM therapy (such as a physician-acupuncturist needling a patient) or a CAM provider (such as a licensed massage therapist) [8]. Hospitals will use credentialing as a baseline attempt to ensure that collaborating CAM providers (e.g., the acupuncturist in the Pain department) are sufficiently qualified and competent to offer services [1, 8, 9]. The first step in credentialing often involves verifying that the practitioner maintains a valid, current license in the state in which he or she wishes to practice [8]. Licensure itself is not a guarantee of competence, though licensure suggests that the practitioner has passed examinations necessary to demonstrate the level of skill and training required by the state in order to practice the healthcare profession [6, 8]. For example, nonphysician acupuncturists seeking state licensure are required to undergo extensive training and to pass a comprehensive examination, which in many states includes a "skills" component [8].

As discussed below under referral liability, it is important to understand the licensure requirements for various CAM professions when a licensed practitioner refers the patient to, or co-manages the patient with, a licensed CAM provider. The referring cancer medicine specialist should know, for example, whether the nonphysician acupuncturist receiving a referral is licensed within the state, as well as what level of training and skill is required as a prerequisite to such licensure. The literature contains basic information concerning the education and training of the four major, licensed CAM professional groups (chiropractic, acupuncture and traditional oriental medicine, naturopathic medicine, and massage therapy) [8].

Additional legal complications may be present if the practitioner receiving the referral is not licensed and is practicing within a state that lacks legislation authorizing non-licensed practice of the healing arts. Just as the unlicensed practice of medicine is a crime in all states, similarly "aiding and abetting" unlicensed medical practice can also be considered criminal [6]. For example, aiding and abetting unlicensed medical practice could be a concern if a court found that a physician had referred the patient to a non-licensed practitioner who was "diagnosing" and "treating" disease. These terms are broadly defined and interpreted, and their boundaries are unclear [6]. This is not to say that such referrals are inherently and always "illegal," but rather that practitioners should flag this practice as potentially raising a legal issue and consider consulting an attorney. There may in fact be situations, for instance, where it is in the patient's best interest to have a referral to someone such as a Tai Chi or Yoga instructor. Assuming the instructor has solid professional boundaries, exercises good judgment and common sense, watches for contraindications and adverse reactions, and refrains from making medical recommendations or interfering with the physician's medical orders, liability concerns should not unduly deter a sensible referral.

3.2.2 Scope of Practice

Scope of practice refers to the legally authorized boundaries of care within the given profession [6]. State licensing statutes usually define a CAM provider's scope of practice; regulations promulgated by the relevant state licensing board (such as the state board of chiropractic) often supplement or interpret the relevant licensing statute; and courts interpret both statutes and administrative regulations [6]. For example, chiropractors can give nutritional advice in some states but not others, and typically, massage therapists are prohibited from mental health counseling [6].

Scope of practice limitations can create liability issues in cancer medicine, as scope of practice places limits on the modalities a practitioner can legally offer. For instance, some states authorize acupuncturists to offer herbal medicine, while other states prohibit such practices. Exceeding one's scope of practice can lead to charges of practicing other healing arts (such as, medicine) without a license [6].

Some institutions will further limit the practice boundaries of affiliated CAM providers beyond the existing limitations of the practitioner's legally authorized scope of practice [1, 3]. For example, the state licensing statute may authorize acupuncturists to practice herbal medicine, but the hospital hiring the acupuncturist into the cancer medicine department may, as a matter of institutional policy, contractually prohibit the acupuncture from employing herbal medicine. Similar controversies might arise in deciding whether and how to credential physician acupuncturists who may have different or perhaps more limited training (e.g., again a weekend workshop) than the training required for state licensure of practitioners of acupuncture and traditional oriental medicine. As suggested, some institutions may address such issues by either limiting scope of practice beyond what the licensing statute requires or adding training standards as prerequisites to practitioners offering designated therapies within the institution (e.g., requiring that physician-acupuncturists have so many hours of clinical acupuncture theory and practice). Such requirements can also serve as liability management tools [1, 3].

3.2.3 Malpractice

Malpractice refers to negligence, which is defined as failure to use due care (or follow the standard of care) in treating a patient, and thereby injuring the patient. While medical standards of care specific to a specialty are applied in medicine, each CAM profession is judged by its own standard of care—for example, claims of chiropractic malpractice will be judged against standards of care applicable to chiropractic [6]. In cases where the provider's clinical care overlaps with medical care—for example, the chiropractor who takes and reads a patient's X-ray—then the medical standard may be applied [6]. We discuss malpractice in more detail below.

3.2.4 Professional Discipline, Third-Party Reimbursement, and Healthcare Fraud

Professional discipline refers to the power of the relevant professional board to sanction a clinician, most seriously by revoking the clinician's license. The concern over inappropriate discipline, based on medical board antipathy to inclusion of

CAM therapies, has led consumer groups in many states to lobby for "health freedom" statutes—laws providing that physicians may not be disciplined solely on the basis of incorporating CAM modalities [6]. More recently, the Federation of State Medical Boards has issued Model Guidelines for Physician Use of Complementary and Alternative Therapies, reaffirming this same principle, and urging physicians to develop a sound treatment plan justifying any inclusion of CAM therapies (see discussion below) [10].

Third-party reimbursement typically involves a number of insurance policy provisions, and corresponding legal rules, designed to ensure that reimbursement is limited to "medically necessary" treatment; does not, in general, cover "experimental" treatments; and is not subject to fraud and abuse [6]. In general, insurers have been slow to offer CAM therapies as core benefits—largely because of insufficient evidence of safety, efficacy, and cost-effectiveness—though a number of insurers have offered policyholders discounted access to a network of CAM providers.

Healthcare fraud refers to the legal concern for preventing intentional deception of patients. Overbroad claims sometimes can lead to charges of fraud, and its related legal theory, misrepresentation [6]. If the clinician or institution submits a reimbursement claim for care that the clinician knew or should have known was medically unnecessary, this also might be grounds for a finding of fraud and abuse under federal law [6].

3.3 Malpractice Issues in Greater Detail

Malpractice appears to cause enormous concern among clinicians and institutions considering the integration of CAM therapies into conventional medical settings [1,3] and is therefore worth reviewing in more detail. Few judicial opinions address malpractice and CAM therapies; the legal landscape is subject to rapid change as CAM therapies increasingly penetrate mainstream healthcare [11]. Yet general principles from malpractice in conventional care still should apply [12].

As noted, malpractice (or negligence) generally consists of two elements: (1) providing clinical care below generally accepted professional standards, and (2) thereby causing the patient injury. The plaintiff (who is suing) usually hires a medical expert to testify that the defendant physician practiced below generally accepted standards of care. There are multiple possible claims of healthcare malpractice, including misdiagnosis, failure to treat, failure of informed consent, fraud and misrepresentation, abandonment, vicarious liability, and breach of privacy and confidentiality [13].

Of these, misdiagnosis, failure to treat, failure of informed consent, and referral liability are often dominant concerns for clinicians integrating CAM therapies into conventional cancer care. The discussion below focuses on conventionally trained clinicians integrating CAM therapies into cancer medicine, although CAM providers can also be liable in malpractice if they violate their own professional standard of care and thereby injure the patient, or alternatively, fail to refer the patient for conventional care when the patient's condition is deteriorating and exceeds the skill or competence of the CAM provider [6].

3.3.1 Misdiagnosis in Cancer Medicine

Misdiagnosis refers to failure to diagnose a condition accurately, or at all, and constitutes malpractice when the failure occurred by virtue of providing care below generally accepted professional standards, and the patient was thereby injured [13]. A conventional provider who fails to employ conventional diagnostic methods where such methods could have averted unnecessary patient injury, or who substitutes CAM diagnostic methods for conventional ones and thereby causes patient injury, risks a malpractice verdict [13].

Adding complementary diagnostic systems (such as those of chiropractic or acupuncture, either by referral or by using modalities within the scope of one's clinical licensure) is not itself problematic, so long as the conventional bases are not neglected [12]. Similarly, it is not malpractice for a CAM provider to use modalities within his or her legally authorized scope of practice, so long as the provider refers to medical care where necessary and appropriate [6]. For example, it would be perilous to treat headaches as "subluxations" or "displaced *chi*" if the patient turns out to have a brain tumor. Continuing to monitor conventionally (or for the CAM provider, referring for conventional care) may be useful in reducing this liability risk [6, 12].

3.3.2 Failure to Treat in Cancer Medicine

The law does not currently distinguish between medical malpractice in conventional care and medical malpractice in "integrative" care. Although some have questioned whether a "mixed" standard of care should apply in the latter case (i.e., taking into account that the clinician "mixed" conventional and CAM therapies) [11], courts are likely to apply the same legal rule as applied to conventional care: malpractice means providing substandard care and thereby injuring the patient [6, 14]. Thus, it is not the use of CAM therapies that is problematic in itself, but rather inducing the patient to rely on such therapies to the exclusion of necessary medical care where such conventional care might have prevented further harm.

In general, the following framework may help the clinician (or institution) to determine the level of clinical risk, and consequently, of liability risk, and to advise the patient accordingly. The clinician should classify any given therapy (conventional or CAM) used for cancer medicine into one of four regions [12]:

A. The medical evidence supports both safety and efficacy.
B. The medical evidence supports safety, but evidence regarding efficacy is inconclusive.
C. The medical evidence supports efficacy, but evidence regarding safety is inconclusive.
D. The medical evidence indicates either serious risk or inefficacy.

In region A, clinicians can recommend the CAM therapy, as a therapy deemed both safe and effective could be recommended regardless of whether it is classified as conventional or CAM [12]. In A, liability is unlikely, because inclusion of the therapy is unlikely to fall below prevailing standards of care (as it is effective), and unlikely to injure the patient (as it is safe) [12]. A salient example would be use of acupuncture for treatment of nausea following chemotherapy, a therapy that has support in an NIH consensus study. Conversely, in D, a therapy that is either seriously risky or ineffective (and thereby delays curative conventional care) should be avoided and discouraged, whether the therapy is medically accepted, or considered part of CAM [12]. An example might be over-reliance on nutritional care where the cancer has significantly progressed and requires treatment through chemotherapy or radiation.

Many CAM therapies will fall within either B or C, where liability is conceivable but, probably unlikely, particularly in B, where the product presumably is safe [12]. If, however, the patient's condition deteriorates in either case B or C, then the physician should consider implementing a conventional intervention, or risk potential liability if the patient becomes injured through reliance on the CAM therapy [12]. The best strategy in B and C is to caution the patient and, while accepting the patient's choice to try the CAM therapy, continue to monitor efficacy and safety respectively [12].

In cancer medicine, some CAM therapies, such as mind-body techniques, have been shown safe and/or effective for conditions such as chronic pain and insomnia, and thus can be recommended [15]. Indeed, different mind-body approaches may be appropriate for different patients at various stages of care, depending on patient needs. For example, relaxation therapies may be appropriate at the diagnosis stage to address anxiety; cognitive behavioral therapy with focus on active coping strategies, imagery, hypnosis, relaxation, and creative arts during active treatment to facilitate treatment tolerance; meditation, Yoga, and creative arts during recovery to help the patient regain strength and deal with existing issues such as meaning and purpose; support groups and retreats during survivorship to promote health and address fear of recurrence; imagery and hypnosis during palliation to assist with symptom control and/or quality of life; and spiritual therapies (including meditation) during end-of-life care to help with issues of transition and transcendence [16]. Again, as regions A through D represent points on a spectrum of safety and efficacy, the cancer medicine specialist will have to decide whether to recommend such therapies if they are safe and effective, or perhaps even if safe but not conclusively proven effective, depending on the patient's needs and situation, and provided that there is no delay of necessary (curative) conventional care. Put another way, even if overall the evidence of efficacy for therapies in cancer medicine may be less than ideal (i.e., region C), liability is probably unlikely if such therapies are generally medically accepted as the best available, and not known to be inherently unsafe or ineffective. This statement should apply whether the therapy is considered "conventional" or "CAM."

On the other hand, inclusion of some CAM therapies can raise the specter of direct harm from the therapy or from adverse interactions with conventional care, or of indirect harm from diverting the patient from necessary conventional care. For example, some herbal products may contain "undisclosed drugs or heavy metals, interaction with the pharmacokinetic profile of concomitantly administered drugs, or association with a misidentified herbal species" [17]. Thus, the clinician must remain alert to the medical evidence regarding CAM therapies, and particularly herbal therapies which may contain previously unclassified hazards; the categorization of therapies over time into any given region of the framework may change according to new medical evidence [12].

Again, by positing the framework in this way, it becomes clear that determining the clinical risk level, and thereby the level of liability risk and nature of patient advice, applies across the board no matter whether the therapy is labeled conventional or CAM. This even-handedness is consistent with the key recommendation of the 2005 Report by the Institute of Medicine at the National Academy of Sciences entitled, *Complementary and Alternative Medicine*: "The committee recommends that the same principles and standards of evidence of treatment effectiveness apply to all treatments, whether currently labeled as conventional medicine or CAM" [18]. Of critical import in having conversations with patients around the conventional and CAM therapeutic options is the inclusion of other members of the care team, such as a nutritionist, psychologist, nurse and social workers, to discuss the whole panoply of supportive therapies, conventional as well as CAM [19].

The above framework for determining the clinical risk level of a given CAM therapy, and advising accordingly, may need to be slightly adjusted by determining the goal of treatment. Thus, "If the goal is cancer prevention, symptom control, supportive care during and after treatment, or general health maintenance, then the clinical risk level is lower than if the goal is antineoplastic in nature" [5]. This means that the cancer medicine specialist may decide to allow greater leeway for inclusion of CAM therapies that have lower evidence of efficacy (yet do not raise undue safety concerns) if the goal of therapy is not antineoplastic [5]. On the other hand, if the goal is antineoplastic, more studies with higher levels of evidence may be necessary to support inclusion of CAM therapies [5]. It is difficult to pinpoint precisely what level of evidence should justify a recommendation, as opposed to the "accept, caution and monitor" response, although one radiation oncologist (Dr. Matthew Mumber) has proposed a decision tree formulation for integrative oncology, accounting for factors including the patient's clinical situation (e.g., acute versus subacute; disease stage and type; prognosis); specific treatment goals (prevention; supportive care; antineoplastic care); general preventive approach (primary; secondary; tertiary); general supportive care approach (translational versus transformational utility; improved tolerance of antineoplastic therapy; symptom control; general quality of life; end-of-life care); general antineoplastic approach (curative versus palliative), and level of evidence for therapy (including data levels for both safety and efficacy; and risk/benefit ratio) [20].

Within the above framework, recommendations involving herbal products remain problematic, as under the Dietary Supplement Health Education Act of 1994, "dietary supplements"—containing vitamins, minerals, amino acids, and herbs—generally are regulated as foods, not drugs, and therefore can be marketed without prior proof of safety and efficacy [6]. Furthermore, in addition to issues of contamination and adulteration, and lack of batch-to-batch consistency, clinicians have to consider the possibility of adverse herb–herb as well as herb–drug interactions. The literature on efficacy is generally sparse compared to comparable pharmaceutical medications, and issues have been raised about both possible benefit and risk from patient use of dietary supplements (including antioxidants) during radiation or chemotherapy.

Sales of dietary supplements as ancillary to treatment also are especially troublesome [21]. So too are any arrangements whereby clinicians receive any percentage or profit from sales of supplements recommended to patients [21]. Such sales can trigger legal anti-kickback considerations. Sales of dietary supplements also can suggest that the clinician has been not only negligent, but potentially reckless, a higher state of culpability, triggering the possibility of punitive as well as compensatory damages [22].

In addition to legal culpability are ethical questions pertaining to conflict of interest [21]. The American Medical Association has opined that physician sale of dietary supplements for profit may present an impermissible conflict of interest between good patient care and profit, and thus ethically objectionable. Several states have enacted laws limiting or prohibiting physician sales of dietary supplements [21]. Yet another concern is potential discipline by the relevant state regulatory boards—such as the state medical board for physicians, as many of the relevant statues contain generic provisions that allow physician discipline, for example, for such acts as, "failure to maintain minimal standards applicable to the selection or administration of drugs, or failure to employ acceptable scientific methods in the selection of drugs or other modalities for treatment of disease" [23].

3.3.3 Informed Consent in Cancer Medicine

The legal obligation of informed consent is to provide the patient with all the information material to a treatment decision—in other words, that would make a difference in the patient's choice to undergo or forgo a given therapeutic protocol. This obligation applies across the board, whether CAM or conventional therapies are involved [24]. Materiality refers to information about risks and benefits that is reasonably significant to a patient's decision to undergo or forgo a particular therapy; about half the states judge materiality by the "reasonable patient's" notion of what is significant, while the other half judge materiality by the "reasonable physician" [24]. Presumably, materiality in the latter half means evidence-informed judgments concerning what therapies may be potentially useful [24].

The principle of shared decision making takes informed consent a step further, by ensuring that there are not only disclosures by physicians to patients, but also full and fair conversations in which patients feel empowered and participatory [18]. The IOM Report on Complementary and Alternative Medicine encouraged shared-decision as a means of patient empowerment [18]. Updating the patient about changes in medical evidence also is an important part of the informed consent obligation. If the discussion involves an herbal product, the physician should try to deconstruct the notion that "natural" necessarily means "safe" [24–26].

An interesting question is how the law might treat clinicians who fail to make recommendations for patients regarding nutrition, mind-body, and other readily accepted CAM therapies as adjuncts to conventional care. If/as medical evidence begins to show safety and efficacy for such therapies, and these therapies become more generally accepted within the medical community, there may be liability for clinicians who fail to make helpful, adjunctive recommendations involving CAM therapies [6, 27, 28]. The case would likely depend on the court's view of whether the medical profession generally accepted the CAM therapy as safe and effective for the patient's condition, and possibly, as a safer and more effective therapeutic option than the conventional drug or treatment route otherwise prescribed [6]. An example might be a patient treated with adjuvant chemotherapy for breast cancer who develops significant nausea, has an extrapyramidal reaction to Compazine, has to pay out-of-pocket for Zofran, and subsequently learns that acupuncture might have more readily resolved her symptoms [19].

In short, engaging the patient in a conversation about options, and suggesting or agreeing to a trial run with a CAM therapy that may have some evidence of safety and/or efficacy in the medical literature, while continuing to monitor conventionally, is a strategy that can simultaneously honor clinical, ethical, and legal obligations. The IOM Report suggested, "The goal should be the provision of comprehensive medical care that is based on the best scientific evidence available regarding benefits and harm, that encourages patients to share in decision making about therapeutic options, and that promotes choices in care that can include CAM therapies, when appropriate" [18].

3.3.4 Referral Liability in Cancer Medicine

A major concern involves the potential liability exposure for referral to a CAM provider. While there are few judicial opinions setting precedent regarding referrals to CAM therapists, the general rule in conventional care is that there is no liability merely for referring to a specialist. It makes sense to apply this rule across the board whether referral is to a practitioner labeled "conventional" or "CAM" [11].

The major exceptions to this no-liability rule involve a negligent referral (one that delays necessary care and thereby causes harm to the patient—in this case, referral to a CAM provider that delays necessary conventional care); a referral to practitioner that the referring provider knew or should have known was "incompetent;" and a referral involving "joint treatment," in which the referring clinician and the practitioner receiving the referral actively collaborate to develop a treatment plan and to monitor and treat the patient [11]. For example, in the first instance, a cancer medicine specialist or a neurologist who referred a patient complaining of persistent headaches to a chiropractor, but then failed to follow the patient conventionally, might be held liable for a negligent referral delaying necessary medical care, if it turned out the patient's headaches were the result of a brain tumor that should have been diagnosed conventionally. Similarly, referral to a practitioner who makes exaggerated claims and lacks even minimum standards of training and skill might be considered negligent referral to a "known incompetent."

The third exception is the most troublesome, as courts have not fashioned clear standards regarding what constitutes "joint" treatment. The notion of "integrative" cancer medicine suggests a sufficiently high degree of coordination between the referring provider and the one receiving the referral that a court could find the "joint treatment" necessary for shared liability, irrespective of efforts to create legal firewalls [11, 22]. In this regard, ensuring that referred-to providers have competence and a good track record in their area of expertise may help reduce potential liability risk overall [22].

3.4 Some Ways to Help Manage Liability Risks

As suggested, a principal strategy to help reduce liability risk involves paying attention to the therapeutic relationship, as injury to the patient and a poor physician–patient relationship can lead to litigation. Safe practice also includes monitoring for potential adverse reactions between conventional and CAM therapies—such as, monitoring for adverse herb–drug interactions. The few judicial opinions on point suggest the importance of conventional diagnosis and monitoring when CAM therapies are recommended or allowed, as a means of ensuring that patients do not receive substandard care [6, 12]. Continuing to monitor conventionally, and intervening conventionally when medically necessary, means that the standard of care likely will be met, and the possibility of patient injury minimized.

Thus, the physician and patient may wish to try a CAM cancer medicine therapy for a pre-defined period of time instead of conventional care (e.g., acupuncture and hypnotherapy) and return to conventional care (e.g., pain medication) when it becomes necessary. From a liability perspective, the more acute and severe the condition, the more important it would be to monitor and treat conventionally. Another risk reduction measure is the practice of obtaining consultation and documenting this in the patient's record to help establish the standard of care in the community [29], and keeping clear medical records that show how treatment options were discussed and decisions made with patients. Physicians also should familiarize themselves with documentation standards suggested by the Federation of State Medical Board Guidelines and whether these are applicable in their state or home institution.

Finally, there is a legal doctrine known as "assumption of risk" that can, in some states, provide a defense to medical malpractice where the patient has chosen a therapeutic course despite the physician's efforts to dissuade and discourage [22]. Assumption of risk has been allowed as a defense in at least one case involving patient election of a CAM therapy instead of conventional care (i.e., of a nutritional protocol in lieu of conventional oncology care) [30]. In this case (*Schneider v. Revici*), the court allowed the patient's signing of an appropriate consent form to serve as an "express" assumption of risk and therefore a complete defense to the claim of medical malpractice. In another case (*Charell v. Gonzales*), a New York court found that the patient had "impliedly" assumed the risk because she was aware of and voluntarily chose a CAM protocol for cancer care, even without signing the requisite form [31].

Based on these cases, some attorneys might advise physicians to have the patient sign a waiver, expressly stating that the patient knowingly, voluntarily, and intelligently chose the CAM therapy or regimen—for example, energy healing and a nutritional protocol—instead of the recommended conventional treatment. Courts, however, tend to disfavor waivers of liability in medical malpractice cases, taking the perspective that medical negligence cannot be waived away, and that the physician remains responsible for the patient's treatment [29]. Although it is unclear that assumption of risk will inevitably be allowed in some form as a legal defense, the principle of sharing information and having patients specifically acknowledge risks of CAM therapies is salutary. Physicians should engage in clear conversations with patients concerning options involving CAM therapies, as such an approach respects is likely to satisfy informed consent concerns, respect an ideal of shared decision making, and encourage positive relationships that can help mitigate the prospect of litigation.

3.5 The Federation of State Medical Board Guidelines for Integrative Medicine

As noted, the Federation has passed model guidelines for: "(1) physicians who use CAM in their practices, and/or (2) those who co-manage patients with licensed or otherwise state-regulated CAM providers" [32]. These guidelines are not binding, but rather offer a framework for individual state medical boards to regulate physicians integrating CAM therapies. They should be read in conjunction with existing medical board guidelines in the state in which the physician practices, as the guidelines may provide ways for medical boards to think about integrative practices.

The guidelines "allow a wide degree of latitude in physicians' exercise of their professional judgment and do not preclude the use of any methods that are reasonably likely to benefit patients without undue risk" [32]. The guidelines also recognize that "patients have a right to seek any kind of care for their health problems," and that "a full and frank discussion of the risks and benefits of all medical practices is in the patient's best interest" [32]. In trying to assess whether an integrative care practice is violative and should trigger physician discipline, the guidelines ask whether the therapy selected is:

- effective and safe? (having adequate scientific evidence of efficacy and/or safety or greater safety than other established treatment models for the same condition);
- effective, but with some real or potential danger? (having evidence of efficacy, but also of adverse side effects);

- inadequately studied, but safe? (having insufficient evidence of clinical efficacy, but reasonable evidence to suggest relative safety);
- ineffective and dangerous? (proven to be ineffective or unsafe through controlled trials or documented evidence or as measured by a risk/benefit assessment).

The guidelines further provide other requirements, such as that medical documentation include a record as what medical options have been discussed, offered or tried, and if so, to what effect, or a statement as to whether or not certain options have been refused by the patient or guardian; that proper referral has been offered for appropriate treatment; and that the risks and benefits of the use of the recommended treatment to the extent known have been appropriately discussed with the patient or guardian; that the physician has determined the extent to which the treatment could interfere with any other recommended or ongoing treatment [32].

The guidelines also provide that the CAM treatment should:

- have a favorable risk/benefit ratio compared to other treatments for the same condition;
- be based upon a reasonable expectation that it will result in a favorable patient outcome, including preventive practices;
- be based upon the expectation that a greater benefit will be achieved than that which can be expected with no treatment.

Again, the guidelines are suggestive but not binding in any given state, unless adopted by that state's medical board.

3.6 A Broader Ethical Analysis

In general, integrative care suggests a balancing of three major ethical values: beneficence (the obligation to help the patient), non-maleficence (the obligation to "do no harm"), and autonomy (the obligation to honor a patient's freely made medical choices) [6]. CAM therapies have forced the medical community to confront a historic position of medical paternalism that insists on doing no harm to the detriment of patient autonomy interests [6]. Thus, if a CAM therapeutic intervention actually succeeds in helping a patient in pain, such an intervention may satisfy the three ethical values above, even if the literature regarding the therapy's efficacy may be sparse.

The approach to ethical decision making based on balancing concerns for beneficence, non-maleficence, and autonomy is found in application of the informed consent doctrine to choices involving CAM therapies. As suggested earlier, the legal requirement of informed consent obligates the clinician to disclose to the patient all material treatment possibilities, including CAM therapies that have some evidentiary support, and to discuss, in a process of shared decision making, potential risks, benefits, and unknowns.

Generally speaking, while the above approach provides a useful guide, it is not enough in light of the historical tendency to dichotomize "conventional" and

"CAM" care and to use the language of ethics as a label for choices not favored by generally accepted conventional models of care. Today, the ethical choices are more complicated than labeling the provision of certain CAM therapies "unethical" simply because the evidence base is not as satisfactory as may exist for some standard therapies. Moreover, the borderline between "conventional" and "CAM" therapies may be difficult to detect [7]. For example, allied health providers such as physical and occupational therapists may offer the patient non-opioid alternatives to cancer medicine that are still considered to fall within the framework of a standard pain practices; they may also offer services such as Therapeutic Touch, Reiki, and other modalities generally denoted as "energy healing" [14], looking for subtle cues to patient improvement even if the medical literature does not definitively conclude whether such techniques have efficacy. It can be difficult, but not impossible, for institutions to credential such practitioners and allow these therapies, and still ensure that the boundaries of professional practice are respected—for example, limiting practitioner claims and patient expectations, honoring whatever contraindications may exist, and referring back for conventional cancer medicine (or other monitoring and care) when necessary [1–3, 14].

More generally, the literature offers one way to break the ethical/unethical dichotomy by instead asking the clinician to review at least seven factors in assessing the ethics of whether or not to offer the patient CAM therapies [27, 28]:

- Severity and acuteness of illness.
- Curability with conventional treatment.
- Invasiveness, toxicities, and side effects of conventional treatment.
- Quality of evidence of safety and efficacy of the CAM treatment.
- Degree of understanding of the risks and benefits of conventional and CAM treatments.
- Knowing and voluntary acceptance of those risks by the patient.
- Persistence of patient's intention to utilize CAM treatment.

The above factors dovetail with the liability approach described earlier. Thus, if the illness is not severe or acute, and not easily curable with conventional treatment, and/or the conventional treatment is invasive and carries toxicities or side effects that are unacceptable to the patient, then, assuming the CAM therapy is not proven unsafe or ineffective, it may be ethically compelling to try the CAM approach for a limited period of time, while monitoring conventionally [27,28]. The ethical posture is even further improved if the patient understands the risks and benefits, is willing to assume the risk of trying such an approach, and insists on this route. In this case, a monitored, "wait-and-see" approach respects the patient's autonomy interest, while satisfying the clinician's obligation to do no harm [27,28].

For example, the use of hypnotism in an effort to reduce the need for painkillers and anesthesia, and to reduce anxiety would, if safe and effective, be ethically compelling, assuming the clinician held a full and fair conversations with the patient about the potential benefits and risks of such an approach. In similar fashion, conversations about the possibility of acupuncture to relieve chronic pain would likely be warranted under the above ethical analysis.

The Institute of Medicine report [18] cited the above ethical framework with approval and highlighted five ethical values to be held in balance in public policy conversations about integration of CAM therapies: a social commitment to public welfare; a commitment to protect patients and the public from hazardous health practices; a respect for patient autonomy; recognition of medical pluralism ("acknowledgement of multiple valid modes of healing"); and public accountability [18]. Regarding the latter, the IOM Report states that some CAM therapies "may have less kinship with technologically oriented, biomedical interventions and greater kinship with therapies at the borderland of psychological and spiritual care that are offered in professions such as pastoral counseling and hospice" [18].

These two new articulated values—medical pluralism and public accountability—enrich the sphere of clinical judgment by adding broader considerations that touch on healing as well as cure. Thus, one can describe a difference between translation of a CAM intervention into a specific desired outcome and use of a CAM therapy to facilitate transformation, defined as opening up "the possibility of seeing the world from a new frame of reference" [5].

For example, many CAM therapies, particularly in the mind-body arena, are generally directed toward transformation rather than translation. Examples might be use of Therapeutic Touch, Reiki, and Healing Touch not only to improve quality of life, including levels of pain, vitality, and physical functioning among breast cancer patients [33, 34], but also to increase the sensation of well-being (e.g., pain, nausea, depression, anxiety, shortness of breath, activity, appetite, relaxation, and inner peace) in persons with terminal cancer [35, 36]. Spiritual care in integrative oncology (including emphasis on search for meaning; "opportunity to move from doing to being;" "connectedness;" and "sacredness of healing") [18] would probably also reflect the ethical values of medical pluralism and public accountability articulated within the IOM report.

In establishing the practitioner's legal responsibilities toward patients interested in integration of CAM therapies (i.e., through scope of practice, malpractice, and professional disciplinary rules), the regulatory structure arguably is moving to reflect this emphasis [14]. Similarly, to the extent that CAM therapies are used for supportive goals (e.g., guided imagery to help with existential concerns during palliative or end-of-life care), the ethical emphasis on values such as autonomy and pluralism may suggest emphasizing transformation over transformation.

3.7 Conclusion

Medical evidence regarding safety and efficacy is in flux, and both medical research and legislative developments reflect a shifting environment for integrative cancer medicine. A stated ideal is to respond to patient interest in CAM therapies in a way that is "clinically responsible, ethically appropriate, and legally defensible" [37]. This can be done by assessing the literature and then determining whether to recommend, approve, or avoid and discourage a given CAM therapy; by asking ask patients, as part of the medical history, what dietary supplements and other CAM therapies they are currently using; by evaluating the extent to which such concurrent regimens may either accelerate or interfere with conventional care; by discussing risks, benefits, and unknowns; and by then advising the patient accordingly within a framework of shared decision making. Finally, clinicians should bear in mind that while legal issues can shape clinical practice, but fear nor ignorance should govern one's view of legal risk; that mitigation of risk and clinical common sense tend to go hand-in-hand; and that depending on the goals of therapy, application of risk management principles can include that notion some CAM therapies can be viewed from the perspective of transformation as well as translation.

Acknowledgments This paper was supported by grants from the Helen M. and Annetta E. Himmelfarb Foundation and the Frederick S. Upton Foundation to the Institute for Integrative and Energy Medicine. While some of this chapter reflects the latest thinking, parts of the legal analysis have appeared in a variety of publications in numerous forms, with detail pertaining to particular medical specialties. The overall analysis also relies the three academic texts cited as original, primary sources and written previously by the author [6, 14, 22].

References[1]

1. Cohen MH, Ruggie M. Overcoming legal and social barriers to integrative medicine. Med Law Int 2004:6:339–393.
2. Cohen MH. Negotiating integrative medicine: a framework for provider-patient conversations. Negotiation J 2004;30:3:409–433.
3. Cohen MH, Ruggie M. Integrating complementary and alternative medical therapies in conventional medical settings: legal quandaries and potential policy models. Cinn L Rev 2004; 72:2:671–729.
4. Mumber MP. Principles of integrative oncology. In Integrative oncology: principles and practice. Oxford: Taylor and Francis Publishing (Mumber, MP, editor), 2005, pp. 3–13.
5. Cohen MH. Complementary and alternative medicine: legal boundaries and regulatory perspectives. Baltimore: Johns Hopkins University Press, 1998.
6. Cohen MH. Healing at the borderland of medicine and religion: regulating potential abuse of authority by spiritual healers. J Law Relig 2004;18:2:373–426.
7. Eisenberg DM, Cohen MH, Hrbek A, Grayzel J, van Rompay MI, Cooper, RA. Credentialing complementary and alternative medical providers. Ann Intern Med 2002;137:965–973.
8. Cohen MH, Sandler L, Hrbek A, Davis RB, Eisenberg DM. Policies pertaining to complementary and alternative medical therapies in a random sample of 39 academic health centers. Altern Ther Health Med 2005;11:1:36–40.
9. Federation of State Medical Boards, Model Guidelines for Physician Use of Complementary and Alternative Therapies in Medical Practice (available at www.fsmb.org, accessed 02/05/04).
10. Studdert, DM et al. Medical malpractice implications of alternative medicine. JAMA 1998; 280:18:1620–1625.
11. Cohen MH, Eisenberg DM. Potential physician malpractice liability associated with complementary/integrative medical therapies. Ann Intern Med 2002;136:596–603.

---

[1] Future legal and regulatory updates and related resources may be found on the Complementary and Alternative Medicine Law Blog (http://www.camlawblog.com).

12. Schouten, R and Cohen MH. Legal issues in integration of complementary therapies into cardiology. In: Frishman WH, Weintraub MI, Micozzi MS, editors. Complementary and integrative therapies for cardiovascular disease. Elsevier 2004, pp. 20–55.
13. Cohen MH. Future medicine: ethical dilemmas, regulatory challenges, and therapeutic pathways to health and healing in human transformation. Ann Arbor: University of Michigan Press, 2003.
14. NIH Technology Assessment Statement. Integration of Behavioral and Relaxation Approaches into the Treatment of Chronic Pain and Insomnia. 1995. Bethesda, National Institutes of Health. NIH Pub #PB96113964.
15. Carlson LE and Shapiro SL. Mind-body interventions. In: Integrative oncology: principles and practice. Oxford: Taylor and Francis Publishing (Mumber, MP, editor), 2005, pp. 183–189.
16. Isnard Bagnis C, Deray G, Baumelou A, Le Quintrec M, Vanherweghem JL. Herbs and the kidney. Am J Kidney Dis 2004 Jul;44:1:1–11.
17. Institute of Medicine (Board on Health Promotion and Disease Prevention), Complementary and Alternative Medicine in the United States (National Academies Press, 2005).
18. Cohen MH and Rosenthal D. Legal issues in integrative oncology. In: Integrative oncology: principles and practice. Oxford: Taylor and Francis Publishing (Mumber, MP, editor), 2005, pp. 101–120.
19. Mumber MP. Clinical decision analysis. In: Integrative oncology: principles and practice. Oxford: Taylor and Francis Publishing (Mumber, MP, editor), 2005, pp. 145–147.
20. Dumoff, A. Medical Board prohibitions against physician supplements sales. Alternative/Complementary Therapies 2000;6:4:226–236.
21. Cohen MH. Beyond complementary medicine: legal and ethical perspectives on health care and human evolution. Ann Arbor: University of Michigan Press, 2000, pp. 47–58.
22. Ohio Rev. Code Ann. § 4731.22 (18).
23. Ernst EE, Cohen MH. Informed consent in complementary and alternative medicine. Arch Intern Med 2001;161:19:2288–2292.
24. Ernst E. Second thoughts about safety of St John's wort. Lancet 1999;354:2014–16.
25. Fugh-Berman A. Herb–drug interactions. Lancet 2000;355:134–138.
26. Piscitelli SC, Burstein AH, Chaitt D, Alfaro RM, Falloon J. Indinavir concentrations and St John's wort. Lancet 2000;355:547-48.
27. Moore v. Baker, 98 F.2d 1129 (11th Cir. 1993).
28. Adams KE, Cohen MH, Jonsen AR, Eisenberg DM. Ethical considerations of complementary and alternative medical therapies in conventional medical settings. Ann Intern Med;2002;137:660–664.
29. Tunkl v. Regents of the Univ. of Calif., 383 Pacific Reporter 2d 441 (Cal. 1963).
30. Schneider v. Revici 817 Federal Reporter 2d 987 (2d Cir. 1987).
31. Charell v. Gonzales, 660 New York Supplement 2d 665, 668 (S.Ct., N.Y. County, 1997), affirmed and modified to vacate punitive damages award, 673 New York Supplement 2d 685 (App Div., 1st Dept., 1998), reargument denied, appeal denied, 1998 New York Appellate Division LEXIS 10711 (App. Div., 1st Dept., 1998), appeal denied, 706 Northeastern Reporter 2d 1211 (1998).
32. Federation of State Medical Boards, Model Guidelines for Physician Use of Complementary and Alternative Therapies in Medical Practice (available at http://www.fsmb.org).
33. Clewell S, Energy medicine. In: Integrative oncology: principles and practice. Oxford: Taylor and Francis Publishing (Mumber, MP, editor), 2005, pp. 425–426.
34. DeVita VJ, Hellman S, Rosenberg S. Cancer principles and practice of oncology. 5th ed. Philadelphia: Lippincott-Raven, 1997, pp. 1541–1616.
35. Clewell S, Energy medicine. In: Integrative oncology: principles and practice. Oxford: Taylor and Francis Publishing (Mumber, MP, editor), 2005, pp. 341–366.
36. Giasson M, Bouchard L. Effect of therapeutic touch on the well-being of persons with terminal cancer. J Holist Nurs 1998;16:393–398.
37. Cohen MH. Legal issues in integrative medicine: a guide for clinicians, hospitals, and patients. National Acupuncture Foundation, 2005.

Chapter 4
Communicating with Patients about the Use of Complementary and Integrative Medicine in Cancer Care

Moshe Frenkel and Eran Ben-Arye

Contents

4.1	Introduction	34
4.2	Communication in Cancer Care	35
4.3	Communication Between Physicians and CIM Practitioners	39
4.4	Conclusion	43
References		43

Abstract Communication is crucial to establishing trust with patients, gathering information, addressing patient emotions, and assisting patients in decisions about care. The quality of communication in cancer care has been shown to affect patient satisfaction, decision making, patient distress, and even malpractice litigation. Communication is now recognized as a core clinical skill in medicine and in cancer care. In using a patient-centered approach, and open communication can be a base to address complementary and integrative medicine (CIM) in cancer treatment. An approach that involves honest and informed discussion on the use of CIM can empower the patient and can benefit both the patient and physician and is described in this chapter. This approach requires collaboration of patients, physicians, and CIM practitioners as essential element in building effective communication. In this way, physicians can fulfill the roles of caring, comforting, and healing, even when cure is not possible.

Keywords: Integrative medicine · patient–physician communication · cancer care · complementary medicine · patient-centered care.

M. Frenkel
Medical Director, Integrative Medicine Program, M. D. Anderson Cancer Center, 1515 Holcombe Blvd., Unit # 145, Houston, TX 77030
e-mail: mfrenkel@mdanderson.org

4.1 Introduction

During the last two decades, cancer care has been challenged with a call for a more patient-centered and holistic approach, as suggested by Engel's biopsychosocial [1] model and themes of patient centeredness [2], mindfulness [3], psychoneuroimmunology [4], and salutogenesis [5]. Healthcare theoreticians and clinicians have largely replaced the biomedical model with a broad biopsychosocial orientation [1] and developed the concept of "patient-centered care" [2]. Patient-centered care emphasizes the need to include the needs and wishes of patients in their healthcare plans. It acknowledges the web of relationships and contexts within which a patient suffers, encouraging the physician to understand both the disease and the patient. Nowadays, cancer treatment emphasizes not only biomedical aspects of care but also considers issues of life quality and spirituality, especially in palliative care [6].

Contrary to a disease-centered approach, which is currently emphasized in conventional care, the approaches mentioned above represent patient-centered approaches and expand the patient–physician dialog to include quality of life, spiritual, and existential issues. This patient-centered approach is based on the assumption that there is healing value to the patient–physician interaction. This interaction affects the patient and his family, the patient's decision-making process, and the quality of his journey in the healthcare system; it may also affect clinical outcomes [2]. This communication describes a bilateral, humanistic, and affective process in which the physician shifts from treating cancer to treating a person touched by cancer.

In using to a patient-centered approach, physicians should consider the role of complementary and integrative medicine (CIM) in cancer treatment. Many studies have confirmed that a majority of patients undergoing cancer therapy also use self-selected forms of CIM [7, 9], such as acupuncture, herbs, diets and nutritional supplements, relaxation, Yoga and others.

CIM is used by over 30% and up to 83% of patients with cancer [7, 8]. CIM use for cancer treatment is more prevalent among women and is associated with younger age, higher education, higher socio-economic status, advanced disease, active coping behavior, and a change in life outlook and beliefs since the diagnosis of cancer [3, 9–15]. In most cases, CIM users are not disappointed or dissatisfied with conventional medicine but want to do everything possible to regain health and to improve their quality of life [3, 6, 9, 10, 16–19]. Patients may use CIM to reduce side effects and organ toxicity, to protect and stimulate immunity, or to prevent further cancers or recurrences.

This extensive use of CIM can also challenge and frustrate the physician as well as the patient, however; the physician is frustrated with his limited knowledge of CIM, and the patient is frustrated when he cannot discuss CIM with his physician. This bilateral frustration results in a gap in communication, which impacts the patient–physician interaction. This gap in communication may also result from the patient's perception that the physician is indifferent or negative toward CIM [16, 20]. As a result, patients often do not report their use of CIM therapies to their provider [21, 22].

Physicians may also communicate information about effective CIM therapies to patients. This failure of physicians to communicate effectively with patients about CIM may result in a loss of trust within the therapeutic relationship. In the absence of physician guidance, patients may choose harmful, useless, ineffective, and costly non-conventional therapies when effective CIM therapies may exist. Poor communication may also lead to a diminishment of patient autonomy and sense of control over their treatment, thereby interfering with the self-healing response [16, 20].

While scientific and evidence-based thinking is fundamental to contemporary medical practice, patients often do not reason in this way. A physician's failure to recognize this interferes with his ability to address the unspoken needs of patients. Psychological, social, and spiritual dimensions of care may be ignored if physicians cannot adapt to the individual needs of the patient or if they provide care without sensitivity. When physicians are faced with unfamiliar information about CIM therapies, they may feel "de-skilled" by being forced outside their zone of comfort and competence. This discomfort can lead to defensiveness and a breakdown in communication with the patient. In contrast, the physician who is receptive to patient inquiries and aware of subtle, nonverbal messages can create an environment in which a patient feels protected [20, 23] and can openly discuss potential CIM choices.

This chapter will focus on patient–physician–CIM practitioner communications related to CIM use during cancer care and recommend an approach for physicians to encourage a successful therapeutic relationship with patients who request advice about the use of CIM in their struggle to overcome cancer.

4.2 Communication in Cancer Care

Communication is defined as the giving or exchange of information, but patient–physician communication is instead not unilateral and is not limited to the transferring of information. Communication is an interactive process. Communication is also not a concise, focused dialog of questions and answers. Patient–physician dialog has a much broader meaning. It involves not just "words"; it is also the "voice." Communication can relate to previous visits, family and caregiver involvement, other healthcare providers, and personal and professional experiences of the physician and the patient. Family, employment, emotions, desires and wants, hidden wishes and concerns, health beliefs, and social, religious, and spiritual issues are all part of communication. Communication involves transference and countertransference and verbal and nonverbal cues.

Communication is crucial to establishing trust with the patient, gathering information, addressing patient emotions, and assisting patients in decisions about care. The quality of communication in cancer care has been shown to affect patient satisfaction, decision making, patient distress, and even malpractice litigation. Communication is now recognized as a core clinical skill in medicine and in cancer care [24].

A study at a large oncology center in Israel that surveyed patients and staff found that patients believed CIM addressed psychological distress and spiritual and religious issues more than staff members did. On the other hand, staff members attributed CIM use more to a patient's disappointment with conventional medicine than did the patients [25].

A study of patients and physicians in the United States found that their reasons for CIM use were slightly different. These patients were using CIM as a source of hope and control and a nontoxic approach to treatment. Both physicians and patients agreed CIM could relieve symptoms and side effects, but physicians were less likely than patients to expect CIM to improve immunity or quality of life, cure disease, or prolonged life [26].

Understanding nonverbal patterns, which include voice tone, pitch, timbre, and tempo, together with symmetry and asymmetry of posture and breathing patterns, are vital to communication. When physicians pay particular attention to incongruencies, in which the verbal and nonverbal aspects are not aligned, it can yield valuable information about the underlying concerns, beliefs, emotions, and expectations of patients. This kind of information gets to the root of problems and facilitates their resolution. Unfortunately, although these skills are easily learned, they are generally either not taught or only superficially addressed in the medical curriculum, as will be discussed later [27]. The Toronto consensus statement published in 1991 clearly showed that communication problems in clinical practice are important and common. It also showed that the quality of communication is related to health outcomes for patients [28]. A review of the literature has shown that healthcare professionals' effective communication improves patient health by positively influencing emotional health, symptom resolution, functioning, and pain control [29]. Effective communication positively influences not only the patient's outcomes but also the healthcare professional's function. Cancer clinicians who feel inadequately trained to respond to patients' emotional needs are at an increased risk of burnout [30, 31].

Patients react to physicians in multiple ways that can inhibit or enhance the relationship. Physicians may become overly distant, leading to both physician and patient dissatisfaction, or they can become overly involved emotionally, which can have serious psychological and clinical consequences [32].

Another issue that needs to be addressed is appropriate response to patient emotions. One of the most challenging tasks in cancer care is determining how to provide an adequate emotional support [33, 34]. An approach that incorporates empathy, friendliness, listening, and humor, that encourages questions, and that checks a patient's understanding of the answers can be helpful.

The issues of CIM use among patients surfaces quite frequently, and clinicians need to develop an empathic communication strategy that addresses patients' needs. This strategy needs to be balanced between clinical objectivity and bonding with the patient. This approach can benefit both the patient and the healthcare provider. Because of the threat posed by cancer and the uncertain outcome of treatment, most patients require much information about their disease and its treatment [35]. As such, patients need reliable information on CIM and easy access to sources about it.

Patient–physician communication is complicated. The use of CIM by the patient may cause additional confusion. CIM is considered to be outside the boundaries of conventional care, and as such, patients may be hesitant to discuss its use. Some

CIM therapies are being administered by a CIM practitioner. This can complicate communication even more because of a triangular relationship: the patient and his physician, the patient and his CIM practitioner, and the physician and the CIM practitioner. A productive and fruitful communication process requires all three relationships to be addressed.

4.2.1 The Patient's Perspective

The patient's perspective is crucial to the triangular dialog between the patient, his physician, and the CIM practitioner. In a study done in Canada with breast cancer patients who used CIM, patients rated their CIM practitioners higher than their physicians in providing emotional support and listening; at the same time, they trusted their conventional doctors more with regard to telling the truth and having up-to-date knowledge [36]. These findings suggest that patients are looking for two complementary qualities of care that each discipline contributes differently to patient needs.

Patients frequently see CIM as a means of taking control over their health and increasing their quality of life [9, 37]. A study performed at the Royal Homeopathic Hospital in London, which offers complementary therapies as part of the National Health System in the United Kingdom, found that the anticipation of psychological support is one of the notable reasons for CIM use among patients with cancer [38]. Studies performed in outpatient oncology clinics in the United States and Switzerland have found the main reasons for CIM use to be the desire to do everything possible to regain health and to feel hopeful [17]. Other reasons were a desire to gain more control in the decision-making process, the use of one's psychological forces, to enhance the immune system, and to use less toxic treatments. In several studies, CIM users expected CIM to improve their quality of life rather than cure the cancer [19, 38]. Moreover, a large study in Israel found an association between recent use of CIM and a change in outlook and beliefs since becoming ill [13].

Several studies have concluded that disappointment or dissatisfaction with conventional medicine does not cause patients to use CIM [18]. Most patients who use CIM for cancer treatment view it as complementary rather than alternative [7]. In one study, 85% of the participants indicated that CIM should be offered at a cancer center as part of the oncology treatment [39].

Even though most patients indicate that they would prefer to get a physician's referral to use CIM [39], in actuality, the majority do not consult with their physician before their decision to use CIM [22, 40]. This is because many patients believe that the physician has limited knowledge of CIM and has no interest in discussing its use. Some feel that physicians' emphasis on scientific studies and evidence-based medicine, rather than patient preferences, is a barrier to openly discussing CIM [16, 20]. However, patients expect their physicians to study the use of CIM specific to their situation, so they can obtain educated advice and collaboration in decision making [9, 37]. If their physicians are not responsive and are not a reliable source of information, patients obtain and collect information on CIM from a variety of other sources, such as friends and relatives, non-professional literature, popular magazines, journals, daily newspapers, the internet, advertisements, and the health food store. At times, this information is inaccurate, and occasionally, it may lead a patient to use therapies that could even be dangerous [11, 41].

4.2.2 The Physician's Perspective

The physician faces multiple questions and challenges when treating a cancer patient who is using CIM, the most important of which are the safety and efficacy of the CIM therapy [7, 42]. Often, no adequate studies of a particular CIM treatment have been reported. However, in recent years, there has been a small developing body of information that supports the use of CIM as supportive and complementary to conventional care [8].

Another challenge that physicians face is not being aware of the prevalence of use of CIM. Studies have pointed out that physicians lack knowledge about CIM and are not sufficiently aware of the number of their patients who are using it [43, 44]). Physicians at a major oncological center in the United States estimated that only 4% of their patients with prostate cancer undergoing radiation treatment had used CIM, when in actuality the percentage was much higher (37%) [23]. Burstein concluded that these and similar findings indicate a "communication gap that separates patient practices from physician awareness" [45].

To address this communication gap, we must look at the medical school curriculum. Exposure to educational initiatives that stressed communication caused students to be more open and able to talk about CIM with their patients and to feel more prepared to treat patients with cancer [46].

A physician should also respect a patient's autonomy and be sensitive to his concerns; this requires a broad understanding of oncological care, especially when one is required to address CIM use. Even though physicians try to base their treatment recommendations on reliable scientific evidence, they cannot overlook the patient's perspective.

Even though discussions of CIM are relatively rare and most likely to be initiated by patients, when the topic is discussed, both patients and doctors say it usually enhances their relationship [47].

In a study of 291 oncology healthcare professionals in the United States, most agreed that good communication enhances patient satisfaction (76%) and treatment compliance (88%). However, only 34% of respondents felt comfortable discussing CIM, and approximately half of all respondents felt they lacked the skills to communicate and help patients maintain hope [48].

A study conducted with German physicians found a different trend. Physicians, particularly general practitioners, showed acceptance of CIM [49]. Approximately half of the respondents supported a cancer patients' desire for a referral to CIM or offered it within their practice. The common reasons for responding to a patient's request were promoting greater patient motivation, enlarging the therapeutic repertoire, believing that CIM could benefit patients more than conventional therapy, and believing that conventional treatment is ineffective in some cases.

4.3 Communication Between Physicians and CIM Practitioners

Another important issue that is rarely presented in the literature is communication between physicians and CIM practitioners. CIM use is usually self-administered, but close to 15% of CIM users see trained CIM practitioners. This may seem like a small percentage, but the actual numbers of visits are high and cannot be ignored. In 1997, it was estimated that the total number of annual visits to CIM providers was 629 million, which exceeds the number of visits to all primary care physicians [50].

To the best of our knowledge, no studies have examined communication patterns between CIM practitioners and conventional physicians. Both practitioners of conventional treatments and CIM need to communicate with each other about the patient's treatment. Opening this line of communication could lead to some positive outcomes: the patient would not feel that he has to keep his CIM use a secret and would be open to discussing it with his physician; the physician would be more involved in decision making about CIM; the CIM practitioner would be viewed more acceptably within the medical community.

Because the treatments can enhance or decrease the effects of the other and could harm the patient, this communication is crucial [51]. For example, at a large oncology center in the United States, 25% of patients receiving chemotherapy were concurrently using dietary supplements suspected to have adverse interactions with chemotherapy [52].

Recently, the conventional medical system is now gradually accepting the idea of adding CIM as an elective topic in medical schools. And it seems that most CIM schools are adding topics to their curriculum related to conventional medicine, such as anatomy and physiology. However, neither school of thought teaches how these therapies can be integrated into the current medical system. As a result, both disciplines are working in parallel lines, but the lines of communication and cooperation do not meet and do not produce true collaboration. A recent study of CIM students found that 74% of the students had difficulty communicating with conventional healthcare practitioners. The reasons behind these difficulties related to a fear of being rejected and feeling inferior to conventional practitioners [53]. In a national education dialog to advance integrated healthcare, it was noted that U.S. CIM providers are also quite dissatisfied with the level of interest in CIM at conventional institutions. They mention a communication gap and an "us and them" mindset rather than CIM providers being seen as an integral part of the healthcare system. They object to CIM simply being an add-on to conventional medical care [54].

Israeli researchers have shown that even when CIM practitioners are on staff at conventional healthcare institutions, they are not truly integrated into the system. Dominant biomedical patterns of professional interaction continue to exist, CIM practitioners are not accepted as regular staff members, and their marginality is made clear by a variety of visible structural, symbolic, and geographic cues [53, 55, 56].

There is thus a major communication gap between CIM practitioners and conventional healthcare providers. Comprehensive educational programs in both disciplines can bridge this communication gap. Communicating with the patient's CIM practitioners and developing a common language could create a multidisciplinary, comprehensive teamwork that can benefit the patient who decides to integrate CIM therapies in his care.

4.3.1 Building the Bridge of Communication

An open dialog between patients, physicians, and CIM practitioners is crucial to bridging the communication gap between them. To be open to the patient's perspective and sensitive to his or her need for autonomy and empowerment, physicians may need to shift their perspectives. Physicians should create an open, trustful dialog by simply asking the patient about CIM use and being willing to respectfully listen to the answer, without prejudice and judgment. Today's informed patients value physicians who appreciate them as empowered participants in their own healthcare choices. The physician or other healthcare provider is an informed intermediary, an expert guide, a consultant. Ultimately, the patient might be encouraged and supported to make his or her own choices, informed by the best knowledge of the doctor. It is also appropriate for the physician to raise the question of CIM use with patients and for the patient and physician to decide together on therapeutic management options at each stage of cancer care, from prevention to acute active care (radiation, chemotherapy, and surgery) and to post-acute care (follow-up visits and prevention of recurrence). The main purpose of the patient–physician discussion is not to prove or disprove the efficacy of CIM treatments but to sharpen and refine the questions that might come up when faced with uncertain information about therapies. We believe that asking the right questions, particularly when final answers are not available, will lead to improved patient–physician communication and a rational strategy to address patients' needs and expectations in the face of uncertainty.

To help cancer patients be truly informed and autonomous, physicians need to do the following:

1. Identify the patient's beliefs, fears, hopes, expectations, and experience with CIM.
2. Learn what conventional treatments have been tried, have failed, or have been rejected because of safety, quality of life, cost, or other issues.
3. Make sure the patient understands prognostic factors associated with his stage of the disease and the potential risks and benefits of conventional therapy.
4. Acknowledge the patient's spiritual and religious values and beliefs, including views about quality of life and end-of-life issues, and seek to understand how these impact healthcare choices.
5. Discover what levels of support the patient relies on from family, community, faith, and friends [57].

Before physicians can assess the value of specific CIM therapies, they must determine why the patient is seeking them. Is the use of CIM related to a patient's uneasiness or ambivalence about conventional options? Is it because of a fear of side effects or a feeling that therapy is not working, or is it just to improve and support the conventional treatment? Is the patient looking for a different quality of therapeutic interaction and care and for more individualized holistic care, or are there other issues at play that were not disclosed during the regular visit with the physician? At times, it is not the patient that initiates CIM use but a close friend or a family member; in these situations, it might be important to involve that person in the discussion as well.

By creating a trusting relationship based on good patient–physician communication, misunderstandings can be avoided [12, 58]. Perhaps, the optimal approach is to discuss the facts and the uncertainty with the patient in order to reach a mutually informed decision about the patient's care [13, 59].

Communicating and collaborating with CIM practitioners is another essential part of integrating CIM into a successful patient care plan. Working as a multidisciplinary team by consulting with each other openly and maintaining high degree of professionalism will work to the patient best interests. Putting forth an effort to improve dialog and communication can overcome the Tower of Babel effect [60] a common situation in which the two schools of thought, conventional medicine and CIM, are talking in two separate languages, and one cannot understand the other. Overcoming this communication gap can lead to learning a common language and to a true collaboration.

4.3.2 A Suggested Approach

From the perspective of evidence-based medicine, a physicians' review of the current literature is often not sufficient to answer questions about CIM with a high level of certainty. So the challenge for the clinician is how to deal with an issue that has a high level of uncertainty. Physicians urgently need to approach CIM use in cancer in a systematic way. Occasionally, there is scientific data, though limited, in the medical literature that support the use of CIM, even though they cannot be considered proofs of efficacy; but at times, the data do offer clinical clues that support the use or avoidance of specific CIM therapies. Clues, such a small cohort study, pilot studies, epidemiological data, and others, can provide a basis for honest and open discussion with the patient.

We suggest a rational strategy for approaching CIM use (Fig. 4.1). The first step is for the physician to increase his knowledge about the treatment in question, mainly by searching reliable web sites [61–63] as well as Medline. Ignorance of CIM is no longer excusable, as information is widely available in medical journals, texts, reliable web sites, and databases. *Primum non nocere* is the dictum of physicians: first of all, to do no harm. A corollary to this dictum may be stated as "prevent the patient from harming himself." The doctor has to examine two main issues: safety and efficacy. In examining the safety of the treatment, a physician must consider its side-effect profile and possible interactions with other treatments.

It is necessary for the doctor to frankly and non-judgmentally discuss the known risks and benefits of these CIM supplements with the patient. No matter how safe a therapy is, if it is ineffective, the patient must be informed. CIM therapies, by

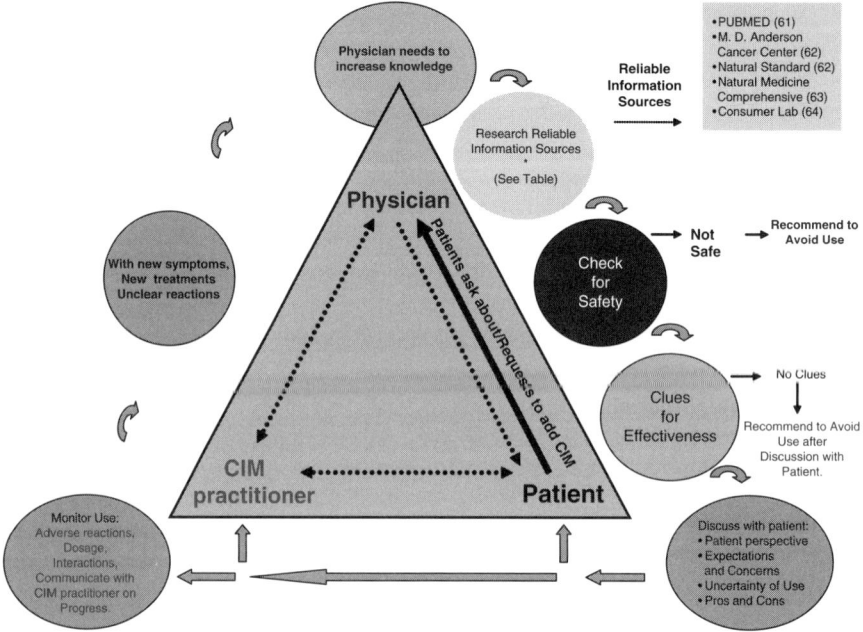

Fig. 4.1 Strategy for Approaching the Use of CIM by cancer patients

definition, have generally not reached the level of evidence of many conventional therapies. They exist at the interface of science and healing. However, many cancer therapies, including chemotherapy, radiation therapy, and a number of plant-based agents, were also considered "alternative" before they were accepted as the standard of care. Moreover, arguing that patients should not try an unproven therapy that they are convinced will be helpful is not very productive. In fact, it is likely to damage the therapeutic relationship and thwart the communication process. It may even be considered cruel; if no better conventional therapy is available.

If it seems that a CIM therapy is safe and there are clinical clues that it may have some effectiveness, the next step is to discuss the level of uncertainty of the treatment with the patient. A physician may tell the patient that more complete information is not available and that a decision about CIM use needs to balance risk and benefit. The higher the patient's expectations, the greater the disappointment when the course of care does not go as expected. As such, the doctor should provide basic hard data on the supplement in order to minimize unrealistic expectations. This discussion can also be used as a tool to improve patient–physician communication and empower the patient in his own care.

If a decision is reached to add a CIM therapy to the conventional treatment of cancer, it does not mean that the physician's role has ended. If the CIM therapy is a commercial product, the physician still has the responsibility of verifying, with some degree of certainty, the reliability and quality of the product (active ingredients, standardization, and so on). A physician with some market knowledge can verify a product's reliability by checking independent web sites [64]. Once product selection and dosage are determined, regular follow-up is needed to monitor adverse effects and effectiveness and to make dosage adjustments, as with any medication.

If the CIM treatment selected requires professional intervention, the next step is to find the right CIM provider. Patients need to consider the practitioner's accessibility, length of an average treatment session, cost, and the expected number of treatment sessions. An important part of this selection process is the verification of the professional background of the CIM provider. In the United States, more states are beginning licensure for CIM providers. Recent guidelines released by The Federation of State Medical Boards of the United States suggest that referrals be made to licensed or otherwise state-regulated healthcare practitioners with the requisite training and skills to utilize the CIM therapy being recommended [65]. In those regions where licensure is not required, one can consider the school that the practitioner attended, duration of study, certification, and membership in a professional society. In addition, recommendations from patients and professional colleagues are time-honored, even if imperfect.

For the physician, it is essential to work with CIM providers who are amenable to open communication and perhaps even consider the cooperative care of patients. Qualified CIM providers should be able to identify the conditions that would and would not respond well to CIM treatment. At the same time, CIM providers should be able to discuss their limitations in treating patients' medical problems as well as conditions they would feel uncomfortable treating or would refuse to treat. Physicians should develop their own lists of trusted CIM providers that they are comfortable working with; this usually can be accomplished after meeting and screening these providers.

4.4 Conclusion

The role of CIM in cancer care is controversial. There is a high level of uncertainty about its efficacy and doubts about its potentially adverse interactions with conventional medicine. Nonetheless, because of the increased use of these therapies by patients that suffer from cancer, physicians need to take a new approach and to communicate with their patients about CIM. A patient-centered approach that involves honest and informed discussion on the use of CIM can empower the patient and can benefit both the patient and physician. This approach requires collaboration of patients, physicians, and CIM practitioners, as essential element in building effective communication. In this way, physicians can fulfill the roles of caring, comforting, and healing, even when cure is not possible.

References

1. Engel GL. The need for a new medical model: a challenge for biomedicine. *Science* Apr 8 1977;196(4286):129–136.
2. Stewart M, Brown JB, Donner A, et al. The impact of patient-centered care on outcomes. *J Fam Pract* Sep 2000;49(9):796–804.

3. Epstein RM. Mindful practice. *JAMA* Sep 1 1999;282(9):833–839.
4. Prolo P, Chiappelli F, Fiorucci A, Dovio A, Sartori ML, Angeli A. Psychoneuroimmunology: new avenues of research for the twenty-first century. *Ann N Y Acad Sci* Jun 2002;966:400–408.
5. Sagy S, Antonovsky H. The development of the sense of coherence: a retrospective study of early life experiences in the family. *Int J Aging Hum Dev* 2000;51(2):155–166.
6. Rabow MW, Dibble SL, Pantilat SZ, McPhee SJ. The comprehensive care team: a controlled trial of outpatient palliative medicine consultation. *Arch Intern Med* Jan 12 2004;164(1): 83–91.
7. Richardson MA, Sanders T, Palmer JL, Greisinger A, Singletary SE. Complementary/alternative medicine use in a comprehensive cancer center and the implications for oncology. *J Clin Oncol* Jul 2000;18(13):2505–2514.
8. Ernst E, Cassileth BR. The prevalence of complementary/alternative medicine in cancer: a systematic review. *Cancer* Aug 15 1998;83(4):777–782.
9. Crocetti E, Crotti N, Feltrin A, Ponton P, Geddes M, Buiatti E. The use of complementary therapies by breast cancer patients attending conventional treatment. *Eur J Cancer* Feb 1998;34(3):324–328.
10. Miller M, Boyer MJ, Butow PN, Gattellari M, Dunn SM, Childs A. The use of unproven methods of treatment by cancer patients. Frequency, expectations and cost. *Support Care Cancer* Jul 1998;6(4):337–347.
11. Rees RW, Feigel I, Vickers A, Zollman C, McGurk R, Smith C. Prevalence of complementary therapy use by women with breast cancer. A population-based survey. *Eur J Cancer* Jul 2000;36(11):1359–1364.
12. Sollner W, Maislinger S, DeVries A, Steixner E, Rumpold G, Lukas P. Use of complementary and alternative medicine by cancer patients is not associated with perceived distress or poor compliance with standard treatment but with active coping behavior: a survey. *Cancer* Aug 15 2000;89(4):873–880.
13. Paltiel O, Avitzour M, Peretz T, et al. Determinants of the use of complementary therapies by patients with cancer. *J Clin Oncol* May 1 2001;19(9):2439–2448.
14. Edgar L, Remmer J, Rosberger Z, Fournier MA. Resource use in women completing treatment for breast cancer. *Psychooncology* Sep–Oct 2000;9(5):428–438.
15. Alferi SM, Antoni MH, Ironson G, Kilbourn KM, Carver CS. Factors predicting the use of complementary therapies in a multi-ethnic sample of early-stage breast cancer patients. *J Am Med Womens Assoc* Summer 2001;56(3):120–123, 126.
16. Wyatt GK, Friedman LL, Given CW, Given BA, Beckrow KC. Complementary therapy use among older cancer patients. *Cancer Pract* May–Jun 1999;7(3):136–144.
17. Morant R, Jungi WF, Koehli C, Senn HJ. [Why do cancer patients use alternative medicine?]. *Schweiz Med Wochenschr* Jul 9 1991;121(27–28):1029–1034.
18. Kappauf H, Leykauf-Ammon D, Bruntsch U, et al. Use of and attitudes held towards unconventional medicine by patients in a department of internal medicine/oncology and haematology. *Support Care Cancer* Jul 2000;8(4):314–322.
19. Oneschuk D, Fennell L, Hanson J, Bruera E. The use of complementary medications by cancer patients attending an outpatient pain and symptom clinic. *J Palliat Care* Winter 1998;14(4):21–26.
20. Tasaki K, Maskarinec G, Shumay DM, Tatsumura Y, Kakai H. Communication between physicians and cancer patients about complementary and alternative medicine: exploring patients' perspectives. *Psychooncology* May–Jun 2002;11(3):212–220.
21. Fernandez CV, Stutzer CA, MacWilliam L, Fryer C. Alternative and complementary therapy use in pediatric oncology patients in British Columbia: prevalence and reasons for use and nonuse. *J Clin Oncol* Apr 1998;16(4):1279–1286.
22. Von Gruenigen VE, White LJ, Kirven MS, Showalter AL, Hopkins MP, Jenison EL. A comparison of complementary and alternative medicine use by gynecology and gynecologic oncology patients. *Int J Gynecol Cancer* May–Jun 2001;11(3):205–209.
23. Kao GD, Devine P. Use of complementary health practices by prostate carcinoma patients undergoing radiation therapy. *Cancer* Feb 1 2000;88(3):615–619.

24. Baile WF, Aaron J. Patient-physician communication in oncology: past, present, and future. *Curr Opin Oncol* Jul 2005;17(4):331–335.
25. Ben-Arye E, Bar-Sela G, Frenkel M, Kuten A, Hermoni D. Is a biopsychosocial-spiritual approach relevant to cancer treatment? A study of patients and oncology staff members on issues of complementary medicine and spirituality. *Support Care Cancer* Feb 2006;14(2): 147–152.
26. Richardson MA, Masse LC, Nanny K, Sanders C. Discrepant views of oncologists and cancer patients on complementary/alternative medicine. *Support Care Cancer* Nov 2004;12(11): 797–804.
27. Walker L. Non-verbal communication. *BMJ, Rapid responses* [July 6, 1998; http://bmj.bmjjournals.com/cgi/eletters/316/7149/1922#323].
28. Simpson M, Buckman R, Stewart M, et al. Doctor-patient communication: the Toronto consensus statement. *BMJ* Nov 30 1991;303(6814):1385–1387.
29. Stewart MA. Effective physician-patient communication and health outcomes: a review. *CMAJ* May 1 1995;152(9):1423–1433
30. Ramirez AJ, Graham J, Richards MA, et al. Burnout and psychiatric disorder among cancer clinicians. *Br J Cancer* Jun 1995;71(6):1263–1269.
31. Ramirez AJ, Graham J, Richards MA, Cull A, Gregory WM. Mental health of hospital consultants: the effects of stress and satisfaction at work. *Lancet* Mar 16 1996;347(9003):724–728.
32. Farber NJ, Novack DH, O'Brien MK. Love, boundaries, and the patient-physician relationship. *Arch Intern Med* Nov 10 1997;157(20):2291–2294.
33. Buckman R. Communications and emotions. *BMJ* Sep 28 2002;325(7366):672.
34. Tattersall MH, Gattellari M, Voigt K, Butow PN. When the treatment goal is not cure: are patients informed adequately? *Support Care Cancer.* May 2002;10(4):314–321.
35. Jenkins V, Fallowfield L, Saul J. Information needs of patients with cancer: results from a large study in UK cancer centres. *Br J Cancer* Jan 5 2001;84(1):48–51.
36. Boon H, Stewart M, Kennard MA, et al. Use of complementary/alternative medicine by breast cancer survivors in Ontario: prevalence and perceptions. *J Clin Oncol* Jul 2000;18(13): 2515–2521.
37. Eliason BC, Huebner J, Marchand L. What physicians can learn from consumers of dietary supplements. *J Fam Pract* Jun 1999;48(6):459–463.
38. Stevensen C. Assessing needs of people with cancer. *Contemp Nurse* Mar 1996;5(1):36–39.
39. Coss RA, McGrath P, Caggiano V. Alternative care. Patient choices for adjunct therapies within a cancer center. *Cancer Pract* May–Jun 1998;6(3):176–181.
40. Eliason BC, Myszkowski J, Marbella A, Rasmann DN. Use of dietary supplements by patients in a family practice clinic. *J Am Board Fam Pract* Jul–Aug 1996;9(4):249–253.
41. Gotay CC, Dumitriu D. Health food store recommendations for breast cancer patients. *Arch Fam Med* Aug 2000;9(8):692–699.
42. Weiger WA, Smith M, Boon H, Richardson MA, Kaptchuk TJ, Eisenberg DM. Advising patients who seek complementary and alternative medical therapies for cancer. *Ann Intern Med* Dec 3 2002;137(11):889–903.
43. Newell S, Sanson-Fisher RW. Australian oncologists' self-reported knowledge and attitudes about non-traditional therapies used by cancer patients. *Med J Aust* Feb 7 2000;172(3): 110–113.
44. Bourgeault IL. Physicians' attitudes toward patients' use of alternative cancer therapies. *CMAJ* Dec 15 1996;155(12):1679–1685.
45. Burstein HJ. Discussing complementary therapies with cancer patients: what should we be talking about? *J Clin Oncol* Jul 2000;18(13):2501–2504.
46. Ben-Arye E, Frenkel M. An approach to teaching physicians about complementary medicine in the treatment of cancer. *Integr Cancer Ther* Sep 2004;3(3):208–213.
47. Roberts CS, Baker F, Hann D, et al. Patient-physician communication regarding use of complementary therapies during cancer treatment. *J Psychosoc Oncol* 2005;23(4):35–60.
48. Roberts C, Benjamin H, Chen L, et al. Assessing communication between oncology professionals and their patients. *J Cancer Educ* Summer 2005;20(2):113–118.

49. Munstedt K, Entezami A, Wartenberg A, Kullmer U. The attitudes of physicians and oncologists towards unconventional cancer therapies (UCT). *Eur J Cancer* Oct 2000;36(16): 2090–2095.
50. Eisenberg DM, Davis RB, Ettner SL, et al. Trends in alternative medicine use in the United States, 1990-1997: results of a follow-up national survey. *JAMA* Nov 11 1998;280(18): 1569–1575.
51. Meijerman I, Beijnen JH, Schellens JH. Herb-drug interactions in oncology: focus on mechanisms of induction. *Oncologist* Jul–Aug 2006;11(7):742–752.
52. Gupta D, Lis CG, Birdsall TC, Grutsch JF. The use of dietary supplements in a community hospital comprehensive cancer center: implications for conventional cancer care. *Support Care Cancer* Nov 2005;13(11):912–919.
53. Frenkel M, Ben-Arye E, Geva H, Klein A. Educating CAM Practitioners about Integrative Medicine: An Approach to Overcoming the Communication gap with Conventional Healthcare Practitioneres, *J Altern Compliment Med.* 2007 Apr, 13(3):387–391.
54. Weeks J, Quinn S, O'Bryon, Haramati A. *National Education Dialogue to Advance Integrated Health Care: Creating Common Ground:* Progress Report Integrated Healthcare Policy Consortium; 2004.
55. Hollenberg D. Uncharted ground: patterns of professional interaction among complementary/alternative and biomedical practitioners in integrative health care settings. *Soc Sci Med* Feb 2006;62(3):731–744.
56. Shuval JT, Mizrachi N, Smetannikov E. Entering the well-guarded fortress: alternative practitioners in hospital settings. *Soc Sci Med* Nov 2002;55(10):1745–1755.
57. Frenkel M, Ben-Arye E, Baldwin CD, Sierpina V. Approach to communicating with patients about the use of nutritional supplements in cancer care. *South Med J* Mar 2005;98(3):289–294.
58. Sierpina V. Ethics Forum: Complementary Medicine and Cancer Care. *Am Med News*, Oct 4, 2004.
59. Ben-Arye E, Frenkel M, Margalit RS. Approaching complementary and alternative medicine use in patients with cancer: questions and challenges. *J Ambul Care Manage* Jan–Mar 2004;27(1):53–62.
60. Caspi O, Bell IR, Rychener D, Gaudet TW, Weil AT. The Tower of Babel: communication and medicine: an essay on medical education and complementary-alternative medicine. *Arch Intern Med* Nov 27 2000;160(21):3193–3195.
61. University of Texas Medical Branch CAM website. http://cam.utmb.edu/default.asp. Accessed August 12, 2006.
62. M. D. Anderson Cancer Center CAM website. http://www.mdanderson.org/departments/CIMER/. Accessed October 12, 2006.
63. Natural Medicine Comprehensive Database. http://www.naturaldatabase.com/. Accessed August 12, 2006.
64. ConsumerLab.com, LLC. http://www.consumerlab.com/index.asp. Accessed August 12, 2006.
65. New model guidelines for the use of complementary and alternative therapies in medical practice. *Altern Ther Health Med* Jul–Aug 2002;8(4):44–47.

Integrative Oncology Programs at National Cancer Institute Comprehensive Cancer Centers

Chapter 5
The Integrative Medicine Program at The University of Texas M. D. Anderson Cancer Center

Lorenzo Cohen, Laura Baynham-Fletcher, and Catherine Kirkwood

Contents

5.1	Combining the Best Approaches from Conventional and Complementary Medicine	50
5.2	Clinical Delivery	50
5.3	Education	57
5.4	Marketing	63
5.5	Research	64
5.6	Summary	65
References		65

Abstract The Integrative Medicine Program at The University of Texas M. D. Anderson Cancer Center focuses on treating cancer in the whole person. The program has three areas of emphasis: clinical delivery, education, and research. Clinically, we provide the highest quality integrative medicine therapies to patients and their families by using a patient-centered approach. The therapies are provided in concert with mainstream care to manage symptoms, relieve stress, enhance quality of life, and guide patients in their use of complementary medicine. Our educational focus is on providing reliable information on integrative medicine treatment options to patients, families, and medical staff of M. D. Anderson. This is done through our Web site (http://www.mdanderson.org/cimer), a lecture series, development of CD ROMs, and educating the next generation of medical professionals. Our research is advancing knowledge on the outcome and effectiveness of these therapies through peer-reviewed, mixed-methodology research. We are examining treatments to reduce the negative effects of cancer diagnosis and treatment and improving treatment outcomes and quality of life. Starting an integrative medicine program within a conventional medical setting takes careful planning. This chapter presents details on the clinical and educational aspects of M. D. Anderson's program with an emphasis on how we started each, advice to those wanting to start a similar program, and important processes that are in place

---

L. Cohen
Director, Integrative Medicine Program, M. D. Anderson Cancer Center, 1515 Holcombe Blvd., Unit # 145, Houston, TX 77030
e-mail: lcohen@mdanderson.org

to ensure continued success. Collaboration remains the key to the evolving clinical, educational, and research efforts of the Integrative Medicine Program.

Keywords: Integrative medicine · oncology · patient-centered care · education.

5.1 Combining the Best Approaches from Conventional and Complementary Medicine

The Integrative Medicine Program at The University of Texas M. D. Anderson Cancer Center, located in the Texas Medical Center in Houston, centers on treating cancer in the whole person. The program's mission focuses on three areas: clinical delivery, education, and research. The main objectives of these areas are as follows:

1. Clinical: To provide the highest quality integrative medicine therapies to patients and their families by using a patient-centered approach. The therapies are provided in concert with mainstream care to manage symptoms, relieve stress, and enhance quality of life.
2. Education: Offer reliable information on integrative medicine treatment options to patients, families, and medical staff of M. D. Anderson.
3. Research: Advance knowledge on the outcome and effectiveness of these therapies through peer-reviewed, mixed-methodology research.

This chapter will focus on describing the clinical and educational aspects of the Integrative Medicine Program at M. D. Anderson. An interesting aspect of the program evolution is that these two components developed at different times and prior to the formalization of the Integrative Medicine Program, the clinical aspect starting in 1998 and the education component in 2000. They also were housed in different areas of the institution. This allowed each area to grow independently of each other, and then after they were established, they were brought together in 2002 to form what is now the Integrative Medicine Program. The Integrative Medicine Program is housed within the Division of Cancer Medicine that includes all of the medical oncology departments at M. D. Anderson. Below we present details on the clinical and education aspects of our program with an emphasis on how we started each, advice to those wanting to start a similar program, and important processes that are in place to ensure continued success.

5.2 Clinical Delivery

5.2.1 Beginnings

In 1995, 7 years after the first Anderson Network Conference (the Anderson Network is an organization that provides patient-to-patient support), *Living Fully and Beyond Cancer*, the seed was planted for Place ... *of wellness*, the Integrative Medicine Program's center for the clinical delivery of complementary medicine. The Anderson Network Conference covered topics such as nutrition, guided imagery, meditation, and support. The conference committee, comprised of patients and caregivers, said to the Anderson Network director one day, "If we can do this once a year and meet such a critical need, surely we can find a way to have something more regularly offered at the institution." This ignited a spark in the Anderson Network director and furthered the vision that was to become Place . . . . *of wellness*.

Along with the help of the chief of the Section of Psychiatry and others, a business plan was developed with a list of existing programs that could be considered psychosocial, supportive, or complementary to patient care and a three-tier fee structure: programs at no cost, programs at a fee for service, and billable services. The proposal for Place . . . *of wellness* was first presented to an audience of well-established M. D. Anderson faculty. Shortly, into the meeting, a faculty member stood up and said, "I've heard enough." As audience members quickly gathered their belongings in preparation to leave, he continued, "We should have done this long ago." And with that, the implementation phase of Place . . . *of wellness* began.

5.2.2 Developing our Mission and Scope

In developing the Place . . . *of wellness*, it was essential to create a Steering Committee. It was comprised of representatives from all major disciplines and included those who were strong advocates, those who still needed convincing, and still others who would come to be major collaborators after a better understanding of complementary and integrative medicine's (CIM) role in cancer and cancer treatment. This allowed for the identification of challenges and opportunities. It was also important to establish roles and responsibilities of committee members up front. Would members have input but not final authority on policies, procedures, and program offerings? Or would they review all decisions on the table and vote accordingly, regardless of the charge and vision of the principal management team? Our committee included representatives from over 14 departments and clinic areas from Social Work, Chaplaincy, and Psychiatry to Behavioral Science, Endocrinology, Patient Education, Nursing, and others. The first item of business in starting the Place . . . *of wellness* was to develop a mission statement and to establish our initial scope of practice. Our mission statement is as follows:

> Place . . . of wellness is an environment where all persons touched by cancer (patients, family members, and personal caregivers, and friends in their support system and regardless of where they received treatment) may enhance their quality of life through programs that complement medical care and focus on the mind, body, and spirit.

We made a conscious decision not to use the term *alternative therapies*, as it is associated with therapies used in place of mainstream care.

Once we knew whom we would serve, we needed to decide what services we were going to offer and who would provide them. An Advisory Committee composed of patients and family members was formed to provide this valuable input and advise us on how best to market and promote these programs. They were also some of our first volunteers, which was quite helpful with initial big events and special projects. We educated Committee members about the different areas of CIM so that we would all speak the same language when discussing various program opportunities and services. We already had a list of ideas for new services; a list of existing support groups, meditation classes, and educational sessions; and a list of services no longer used because of resource constraints. Additionally, we sent out a request for proposals for services to offer at Place ... *of wellness* to all faculty and staff, which was also an excellent marketing strategy. While some of the ideas we received did not fall under our mission, many did. After soliciting ideas, we received a stream of inquiries from internal personnel and from the community about getting involved with the Place ... *of wellness* and offering some type of program. Many of these initial contacts evolved into programs that we still offer today and others were not appropriate once evaluated within our system.

After receiving proposals for services for Place ... *of wellness*, we formed several subcommittees to manage the following issues: program proposal review and facilitator/practitioner credentialing; registration and evaluation; and legal and compliance. While reviewing proposals, we were also looking for best practices of CIM and contacted all of the comprehensive cancer centers and even several centers that were not affiliated with any medical center. In the spring of 1998, when the planning was taking place, there were no fully implemented CIM programs as part of a cancer center, so we took what seemed to be the best practices and processes from several institutions and weaved them into our existing policy and practice and others had to be developed. It was critical to develop policies and practices in consultation with our institution's financial, legal, compliance, and human resource departments, otherwise we could have ended up with an unsustainable and most probably unbudgeted and unsupported program. Working with these groups also helped to build credibility.

One of the challenges in starting this type of multidisciplinary program is not only to get support from the conventional practitioners but also from the complementary medicine practitioners. We hear many CIM practitioners say, "These therapies [CIM] just don't fall into the realm of the medical model." This, however, is somewhat of a cop-out, and this attitude keeps CIM out of mainstream care. Although in some cases it has taken two or three times as long to implement a service than we anticipated, we have had a sustainable and expanding program since we opened the clinic in the fall of 1998.

We have integrated our programs following the institutional model and it has served us well. For example, one day we received a call from the Medical Staff Office that oversees all clinical programs at our institution, inquiring about the backgrounds of our facilitators and instructors. They had been informed that we had over 100 persons involved with our program and yet none of them had been credentialed. We were able to respond immediately by providing documentation of our process for each individual as well as discussing our various meetings with Legal Services, Institutional Compliance, and even the Medical Staff Office themselves as we developed our guidelines for program development, credentialing, quality assurance, and program evaluation. This process was educational and reinforced that the long road we took to establish the policies and procedures was worth it not just from a compliance standpoint but from a quality assurance, credibility, and patient safety perspective as well.

5.2.3 Screening and Processing Program Proposals

To screen program proposals for services to offer at Place ... *of wellness*, we use a simple form that asks for the following information: facilitator information, personnel involved, program goals/objectives, audience, and program format. We also ask for any supporting documentation regarding the content or the facilitator's experience with the program. The proposals were originally reviewed by a subcommittee, but they are now reviewed by the program management team for consistency with our mission, uniqueness, and logistical feasibility of implementation. If the program idea is accepted, the credentialing process is initiated.

Individual services such as full-body massage and acupuncture demanded a different screening process. We first identified a faculty sponsor or consultant. For example, a faculty physician from Physical Medicine worked with us to develop our full-body massage program and continues to consult for the program today, as does a faculty physician from the Department of Anesthesiology for our acupuncture service.

These two services, massage and acupuncture, required a formal business plan to include space modifications, personnel requirements, and proposed fee schedules. In addition, we consulted with everyone from Institutional Compliance and Legal Services to Financial Reporting and Accounting at M. D. Anderson, many other comprehensive cancer centers, and community-based practices to ensure we were following all formal guidelines regarding participant safety.

5.2.4 Credentialing Process, Programs, and Services

We have a unique process for credentialing facilitators who teach our group sessions and provide individual services. We first identify each facilitator/instructor as either an internal employee or external resource. From there, each facilitator is assigned to one of two credentialing tiers. Tier 1 is for facilitators who are proposing programs that are consistent with their job description (e.g., an advanced practice nurse in psychiatry who wants to provide group therapy). Tier 2 is for facilitators who are credentialed in their content area but it is not part of their M. D. Anderson job description (e.g., a statistical analyst who wants to teach Yoga) or for facilitators who are external to M. D. Anderson. Credentialing and beginning Tier 2 programs require more steps, as our institutional faculty and staff in Tier 1 already have credentials and expertise.

Tier 2 facilitators are asked to submit an application, which includes a facilitator application form, a copy of their degree, a copy of licensure, specialty information (percent of time spent per day/week performing the specialty), two letters of reference, professional liability insurance (establishing maximum and minimum requirements), copies of continuing education credits, and a curriculum vitae or resume. Then, a mentor reviews the application and interviews the applicant. The mentor is an M. D. Anderson faculty or staff member whose expertise is closely related to that of the applicant; if an applicant is accepted into the program, he or she continues to maintain a relationship with the mentor(s). Applicants may be asked to demonstrate knowledge of their subject matter. They will also be informed of the types of specialized screening that registrants of their session may need. For example, movement therapists are mentored through Physical Medicine and Rehabilitation Services. The mentor would discuss with the applicant which adaptations or prohibitive poses such as those that may compress the spine (e.g., headstand or shoulder stand). If all parties want to accept the applicant, we then follow-up by attending any classes he or she may teach, talking with his or her clients as appropriate, and contacting applicable licensing boards, educational institutions, and references. All of these processes are in line with our institutional credentialing and hiring processes for conventional practitioners.

It is important to point out that it is sometimes difficult for community CIM practitioners to transition into an institutional setting. Some CIM practitioners think that the medical establishment should adapt to their needs. Often, CIM practitioners do not fully understand what is necessary to meet institutional requirements, and sometimes, they try to change an established culture overnight or try to work their way around the guidelines. This undermines the whole system. An open two-way conversation at the outset is the best way to avoid these misunderstandings. It stands to reason that practitioners from community settings and entering an institutional setting may feel the need to make a difference and that could be seen as "attempting to change the system" by some or all. CIM practitioners need to practice patience and realize that they and their practice are keys that can open doors to a better understanding regarding patient care. While we are working to develop a common understanding and language among the conventional practitioners and CIM practitioners to form what will come to be known as just simply good medicine, we all have to be willing to listen, observe, and educate one another to work together for the good of patients and families.

As a result of our screening and credentialing process, we now offer over 100 program opportunities at Place ... *of wellness* each month in the following categories: support groups, expressive arts, music therapy, massage, acupuncture, movement (e.g., Yoga, Qigong, Tai Chi, pilates), energy, relaxation/meditation, educational forums, and spirituality. All of these programs are offered at no cost with the exception of full-body massage which is provided on a fee for service basis and acupuncture for which we verify insurance where appropriate and bill. Unlike our acupuncture services, our full-body massage services are for relaxation purposes, so they are not billed to insurance companies. Should a therapist identify a particular issue, such as a rotator cuff or lymphedema problem, we refer the patient to Physical

Medicine and Rehabilitation Services for further assessment. In addition to these services, which are conducted in our facilities, we also serve participants in the inpatient setting, the Ambulatory Treatment Centers, waiting areas, and others upon request. Waiting areas can be places of high anxiety—waiting for results, waiting to start a treatment, waiting to visit a family member who is in the Critical Care Center, waiting for a family member's surgery to be completed, and so on. Having a 10-minute relaxation massage in the waiting area, learning a guided imagery or relaxation technique, or making a paper flower can be of great comfort and support.

It is known that people with cancer use CIM to reduce side effects and organ toxicity, to protect and stimulate immunity, or to prevent further cancers or recurrences. Patients often do not report their use of CIM therapies to their provide [1]. This gap in communication between patient and provider results from patients' perception that their physicians are indifferent or negative toward CIM [2] or from physicians' emphasis on scientific studies and evidence-based medicine, rather than patient preferences. We are addressing this communication gap by providing the patients and their family or caregivers with an extensive comprehensive consultation service. A physician-led comprehensive consultation service addresses patient concerns about CIM therapies and cancer care. The physician reviews all the relevant patient information, information resources related to safe CIM therapies, and others sources. Then a multidisciplinary team including CIM providers also reviews the information, and treatment options are determined. Next, the team communicates with the primary physician who asked for the consultation about the options of care for the patient. The integrative medicine physician then discusses the positive and negative aspects of each CIM option with the patient, and the patient chooses the treatment options they want to pursue and they are followed closely. This new approach is continually being reevaluated because it is a work in progress; further details will be available on our Complementary/Integrative Medicine Education Resources (CIMER) Web site.

5.2.5 Registration and Screening

We made a conscious decision to make registration for Place ... *of wellness* separate from the hospital registration because we did not want any CIM charges to appear on hospital bills. In hindsight, for a number of reasons, it would have been advantageous to tie in our registration with the main hospital's. We have since attempted to do so but have been unable to separate patient demographics and other documentation from the financial information. So for now, we continue with our separate registration process, which includes collecting information about demographics, previous CIM experience, cancer experience, emergency contacts, and how participants learned about Place ... *of wellness*. Participants also complete a release/consent form for treatment and undergo a screening in which they are asked about balance problems, unusual shortness of breath, light-headedness or fainting, fractures, and musculoskeletal issues. Participants requesting massage and acupuncture services undergo a more extensive screening.

5.2.6 Funding

At conferences, we sometimes hear administrators say that they are considering opening an integrative medicine center because the centers seem so lucrative. "Just look at how much is being spent each year on complementary medicine," they say. What they do not realize is that unless you charge for all services, broaden the scope to serve the community for fee-for-service, or sell products, it will most likely not be a revenue leader for the institution. There is nothing wrong with designing a business plan to incorporate these ideas. We, however, have not pursued this avenue. We are fortunate that our institution has chosen to provide the primary funding for our clinical programming. As a state institution, we do have certain expenses for which we cannot use state funds, so we rely on philanthropists and internal organizations through which we can apply for funding for start-up services, equipment, special events, or other expenditures from which states funds cannot be used. We have found that funding opportunities for clinical services and programming are quite limited. Most of our services and programs are for patients with any cancer diagnosis, which further limits funding, as there are foundations that fund diagnosis-specific efforts but do not fund efforts for general cancer populations. Though the revenue we receive from full-body massage and acupuncture services do contribute to our Division, the revenue does not come close to the expenses incurred. As for downstream revenue, we do track referrals made to other services, but several of them are also non-revenue centers (e.g., nutritional counseling, and chaplaincy). Again, we are very fortunate with respect to funding given the generous institutional funding we receive, as the philosophy of our institution is that we are here for our patients and families because it is the right thing to do. We will continue to incorporate fee for service or billing as appropriate when supported by the field.

5.2.7 Other Key Operational Areas

Documentation is an essential part of the delivery of integrative medicine services. Not only is it an institutional policy and a requirement of the Joint Commission on Accreditation of Healthcare Organizations, but it is also an excellent way to educate an institution's clinical personnel about the services provided and outcomes. Our CIM practitioners make notes in the medical records of patients and complete progress notes for non-patients, which are kept in our clinic files.

Participant satisfaction and quality assurance. A pre- and post-program survey has been developed for our music therapy, massage therapy, and acupuncture services. Basic information on common cancer- and treatment-related symptoms are tracked before and after each treatment session (e.g., fatigue, pain, distress, and nausea). In addition, we collect participant feedback for the first six sessions of every new program and then randomly twice per year for an entire month for all programs and services. The most valuable feedback results from asking the question "would you recommend this program to a friend" and asking participants to name three things they liked best about the program, what they would change, and what services they would like added.

5.3 Education

Large surveys of CIM use by patients treated at M. D. Anderson suggest that the majority engage in some kind of CIM practice and that many do not discuss this with anyone on the healthcare team [3, 4]. The most common reasons for non-disclosure were that the patients were not asked about it and that it never came up during their appointment. M. D. Anderson's patient satisfaction survey also suggests that as many as 50% of the patients are not comfortable discussing CIM with healthcare staff.

Medical trainees and faculty are generally not trained to understand, accept, or guide patients on the safe use of CIM in combination with the conventional medicine. Because of the high use of CIM by patients, the lack of communication between patients and healthcare professionals, and the fact that many people get their information from the Internet, M. D. Anderson implemented a CIM-based educational project focused on healthcare professionals in December 2000. The educational component of the Integrative Medicine Program provides concise and authoritative print and Web-based resources, seminars, and workshops on CIM.

5.3.1 Programs

5.3.1.1 CIMER Web Site (www.mdanderson.org/cimer)

In 2001, we moved educational materials from The University of Texas Health Science Center for Alternative Medicine Research Web site, which had not been updated since 1998, to M. D. Anderson's Web site and renamed it the Complementary/Integrative Medicine Education Resources (CIMER) Web site. Its purpose is the following:

> To provide evidence-based information to improve the lives of patients who choose to use these therapies under the direction of informed physicians and to provide educational resources to health care professionals and patients regarding the current understanding of complementary medicine and, where appropriate, to assist in the integration of these medicine and therapies with conventional treatments. Our vision is to discover CAM approaches used by patients, distinguish between harmful treatments, beneficial treatments, and treatments that can be safely integrated with conventional treatments, encourage communication between patients and providers, to educate both health care professionals and patients who need a more comprehensive knowledge base with current and accurate information and promote ongoing professional growth through networking in a setting wherein complementary medicine and conventional cancer treatments can be examined together to enhance lives.

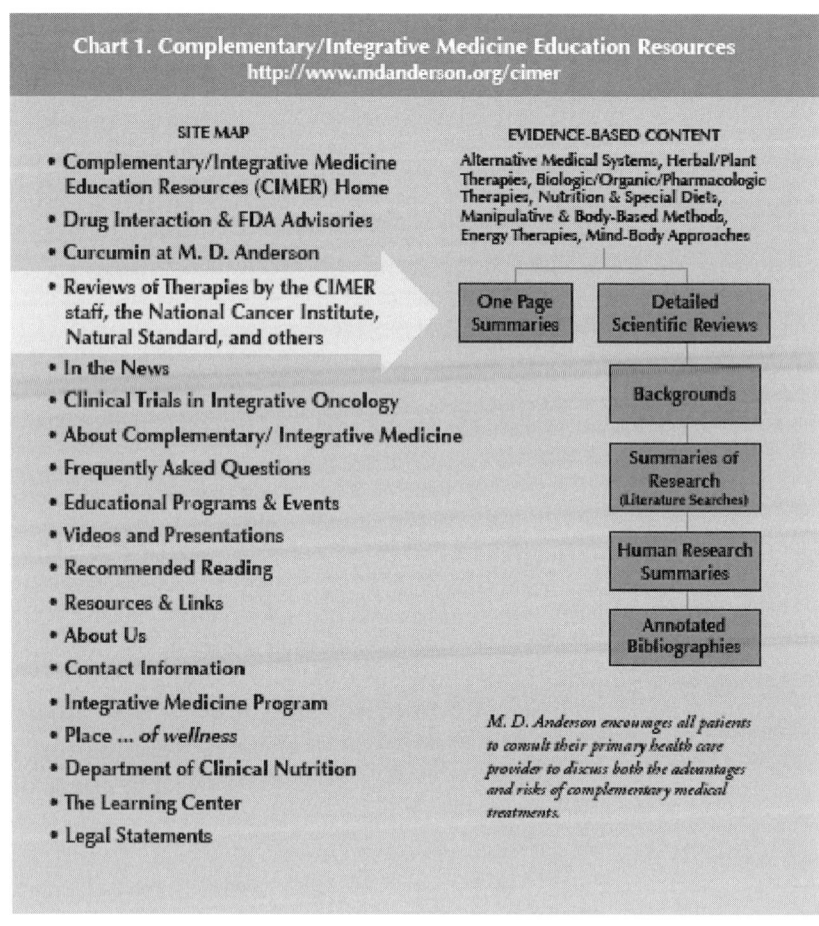

Chart 5.1 Complementary/Integrative Medicine Education Resources (http://www.mdanderson.org/cimer).

In a section of the Web site called "Reviews of Therapies," which is the largest section of the site, we post reviews of various CIM therapies. This section's content is primarily coordinated through our Senior Health Education Specialist and Health Education Specialist who also consult with advisory subcommittees. Other faculty and staff, both internal and external to M. D. Anderson, provide materials as needed and review all materials prior to posting. Chart 5.1 shows the main sections of the Web site. All links are checked at least four times per year to ensure that they are working. The "Videos & Presentations" link consists of presentations by some of our researchers, our communication techniques video series, and our online lecture series.

The Web site has top-level pages in English, Spanish, and Chinese. The Reviews of Therapies section has thousands of structured abstracts and now includes over 80 reviews of evidence of complementary therapies in the following categories:

alternative medical systems, biologic/organic/pharmacologic, nutrition and special diets, herbal/plant, manipulative and body-based methods, energy therapies, and mind/body therapies. Duplication of reviews has been avoided by licensing Bottom Line reviews from Natural Standard and linking to reviews by the National Cancer Institute's Office of Cancer Complementary and Alternative Medicine, the National Center for Complementary and Alternative Medicine, the National Institutes of Health, and the Cochrane Review Organization.

Drug interaction advisories are obtained from the Food and Drug Administration's News Digests. Appropriate resources and links for healthcare professionals, patients, and the public are available on the site from the Cancer Patient Educational Network of the Comprehensive Cancer Centers, the National Cancer Institute, the National Center for Complementary and Alternative Medicine, and other authoritative sources. The "Educational Programs & Events" link includes Continuing Education and Continuing Medical Education opportunities, courses, and events offered both internally and externally.

The Intranet version of the Web site has been developed to be the primary Integrative Medicine Program educational site for faculty and staff. The Web site was developed in collaboration with other departments, including the Department of Academic Programs Educational Products who implement the content; the Department of Internet Services who track usage, implement content, and assist in establishing internal links; UT Television who create streaming videos. Due to overwhelming demand, questions about the Web site and specific therapies are directed to The M. D. Anderson Information Line where staff has been trained by the Integrative Medicine staff to navigate the Web site and assist callers with questions.

The CIMER Web site content policy is that we will draw conclusions only from the most carefully reviewed information available in complete articles published in peer-reviewed journals. Although we note abstracts within the Annotated Bibliography subsection of Reviews of Therapies, we label them as such and do not consider them when drawing conclusions. An exception to this policy is made if an abstract reports the potential harm of using a specific complementary or alternative approach and we believe it is important that such information be disseminated quickly pending further confirmation.

We are very careful not to put anything on the site that is questionable. We only advertise conferences that have speakers who are authoritative, published, and credible in the field. Our goal is to provide only information that is evidence based. We avoid endorsing products and companies.

Because people also use CIM for illnesses other than cancer (high blood pressure, thyroid problems, high cholesterol, etc.), we think our faculty and staff need to also have information about non-cancer complementary and alternative medical (CAM) products. Therefore, each year, we license databases relating to herbs, nutritional supplements, and other CIM therapies.

5.3.1.2 Patient/Provider Communication

The CIMER Web site also includes instruction modules on communication skills for medical professionals and patients. The Web book "Conversations in Care" has a chapter called "The Importance of Physician-Patient Communications" by Dr. Walter Baile, which is linked to the CIMER site. We have also collaborated with Dr. Baile and Dr. Robert Buckman to create video materials to improve communication with patients about CIM. The series of three CD ROMs is called "Important Conversations: Complementary Therapies and Cancer" and is accessible on the Web site. The first CD ROM, "Talking With Patients About Complementary Therapies," approximately 50 minutes long describes CAM and the importance of discussing it with patients. The second CD, "Patients Talk About Complementary Therapies and Cancer," runs approximately 30 minutes and features patients talking about their experiences with CAM. The third CD, "Complementary Therapies: What You Must Ask And Why," runs approximately 20 minutes and features discussions about nutrition; an interview with a pharmacist; legal and ethical issues; and a role-play discussing CIM use. The CD ROM series won an International Health and Medical Media (FREDDIE) Award in the category of Health and Wellness. The series can be viewed for free on the CIMER Web site; the CDs are also available for purchase (the fee covers only the price of packaging and shipping). In addition, this resource is part of the Patient Education Online database at M. D. Anderson, which contains patient education materials that clinicians can print for patients.

5.3.1.3 Lecture Series

The Integrative Medicine Program lecture series is geared toward our physicians, physicians-in-training, nurses, pharmacists, dietitians, physician assistants, and basic science faculty members. It features authoritative speakers from around the world who review and discuss complementary therapies; examining the preclinical and clinical effects of complementary therapies; new drug development from natural products; and research on acupuncture, mind-body medicine, and energy medicine.

Each lecture offers Continuing Medical Education and Continuing Nursing Education hours and our dietitians may apply for credit by submitting a certificate of completion to their accrediting agency. Evaluation forms are completed by participants and reviewed quarterly in order to improve the program and to discover what our participants are interested in hearing more about. All lectures are videotaped by UT Television and some lectures are presented on our Web site or placed in our Research Medical Library. Some of these lectures are available to employees via a CISCO desktop Internet protocol TV (IPTV) system and some are played regularly on 19 flat-screened televisions placed in strategic faculty and staff gathering areas. We also coordinate with Telecommunications Services to broadcast the lectures to several other U.T. institutions and institutions outside the U.T. network. When possible, we share the expenses of bringing in a speaker with other departments or other institutions.

5.3.1.4 Institutional Educational Forums

To provide a forum for CAM education, we participate in other institutional educational opportunities, such as grand rounds. Members of the Integrative Medicine

Program present regularly at division and departmental grand rounds and at the main institutional grand rounds and teach within specific training programs for trainees and fellows.

5.3.1.5 Multi-Institutional CAM Courses

To increase awareness of CAM across the Texas Medical Center in Houston, we have collaborated with other institutions to implement CAM courses. Two introductory overview courses on CAM and one course on the healing traditions from China, Tibet, and India have been taught. The CAM introductory overview course taught at The University of Texas Medical School at Houston has now become an elective offered each year to students and faculty. Instructors for the courses come from M. D. Anderson; The University of Texas Health Science Center's Schools of Public Health, Nursing, and Medicine; Rice University; Asia Society Texas; The Ligmincha Institute; and the American College of Acupuncture and Oriental Medicine.

5.3.1.6 LACE Program (Longitudinal Ambulatory Care Experience)

In the spring of 2006, the Integrative Medicine Program at M. D. Anderson and the LACE Program at Baylor College of Medicine began a collaboration that brings Baylor's third-year medical students in the LACE Program to the Place ... *of wellness* at M. D. Anderson. The students are given an overview of the Integrative Medicine Program and then they participate in program sessions and shadow practitioners.

5.3.1.7 Massage Therapy Course (Massage for the Cancer Patient: An Integrative Approach)

Many Massage Therapy schools still teach that massaging cancer patients is contraindicated rather than teaching how to safely and effectively massage a patient with cancer. It is known, however, that patients with cancer can benefit from massage and some simple precautions and extra training can make it safe to massage cancer patients [5]. The Integrative Medicine Program offers a comprehensive course that trains registered, certified, and licensed massage therapists to work with cancer patients.

5.3.1.8 Research Medical Library

A close collaboration with the M. D. Anderson library ensures that we have appropriate resources on CIM available to faculty and staff. The library maintains video copies of many of our lectures on CIM so that the lectures can be available to faculty and staff. Our Web site and CD ROM series are also available in the library. The library sends us CIM-related books and journals to review. They also track usage of all CIM-related resources and send us a quarterly report summarizing the data.

5.3.2 Internal Collaborations

The development and maintenance of the educational programs are guided by an Internal Advisory Committee of over 20 faculty and staff members from numerous departments who have a special interest in CIM and by a committee of seven external consultants. The Internal Advisory Committee is divided into the following five subcommittees that assist with the following programs: lecture series screening, Web site priorities, conferences and workshops, public inquiry, and Web site reviews. These subcommittees meet only when necessary, and the members are usually contacted with questions or requests for assistance via email. We also have an Operational Committee that assists with internal collaborations and ensures that the program adheres to its mission. These three committees are composed of 47 participants from numerous departments, including representatives from our fellowship programs in Medical Oncology, Radiation Oncology, and Surgical Oncology.

We work closely with M. D. Anderson's Department of Clinical Nutrition, which also provides classes through the Place ... *of wellness*. Each month the department sets up a display of materials on nutrition and cancer in the cafeteria. A third of these displays have been related to complementary nutrition, herbs, phytochemicals, antioxidants, and the therapeutic benefits of functional foods. M. D. Anderson also has a CIM reference center for the clinical nutrition staff to which evidence-based literature and reliable sources of information are continuously added. Our dieticians are competent about herbal therapies because all registered, licensed dietitians are required to complete an accredited, self-study program offered by the American Botanical Council. The clinical nutrition staff educates professionals and patients through presentations and programs at the Place ... *of wellness*, the department of Nutrition internet Web site, and print materials; they also provide clinical training for dietetic interns.

5.3.3 Program Evaluation and Assessment

The impact of the Integrative Medicine Program educational offerings and of Web site usage data is assessed by our Department of Institutional Research and the Department of CME/Conference Services. In collaboration with our Institutional Research Department, we created assessment surveys for our pharmacists and dietitians to appraise critical educational needs. These two groups were chosen because they are most likely to get CAM-related questions from both patients and physicians, and the dietitians in particular have first hand knowledge of what patients are actually taking. Surveys are placed on the Intranet and invitations are sent by email and/or are distributed to them at their monthly meetings. Data from these surveys go directly to Institutional Research and they send us a detailed analysis. The education staff then research the information, prioritize what reviews of therapies are to be completed and placed on the Web site, and decide which continuing education programs should be implemented next.

5 Integrative Medicine Program 63

Our CME office provides a quarterly evaluation report for the Integrative Medicine Program Lecture series, and from this information, we tailor future programs. Evaluations are distributed and collected at all other programs and events such as our massage course, evaluation of the Natural Standard PDA download, and special events. The evaluations are coded by the education staff and sent to Institutional Research where they again provide us with a detailed report. These reports are reviewed periodically and used to improve programming. In addition to evaluating all our internal programs, we also assist in evaluating and planning our external courses with our collaborators at Rice University, Baylor College of Medicine, and The University of Texas Medical School at Houston.

The evaluations and surveys address specific areas of the program as well as overall satisfaction. Areas in which there is less than 85% satisfaction (combined responses of "strongly agree/very satisfied" and "agree/satisfied") indicate a need for improvement or for program review. For some of the programs, we have pre- and post-test evaluations where appropriate that gauge what participants have liked about the program and their pre- and post-course comfort level with the information presented (i.e., after attending this course, how comfortable are you discussing CAM with your patients?), as well as how the information will be used in their clinical, education, and/or research practices. For example, for the CAM courses that are offered in the Medical Center, we administer a pre-course survey, evaluations of each class (each class has a different speaker), and then a post-course survey. We also record various questions that come to us through The M. D. Anderson Information Line, which assists in answering questions from the public about our Web site.

The key to successful education programs is to integrate them into forums that already exist. In this manner, they will not be viewed as alternative but will become accepted as part of the typical, traditional education already provided for faculty and staff.

5.4 Marketing

Effective marketing is critical for the success of any program and especially so for integrative medicine within a conventional medical center. Internal marketing should present an overview of all programs, educational projects, and research to appropriate departments and clinics. We have extensive marketing materials for both our clinical programs and the educational programs. The Place ... *of wellness* has a monthly calendar of services and programs that is regularly distributed inside and outside the institution. The CIMER Web site also has a brochure that we mail internally and externally on a yearly basis along with our CD video series. We also utilize all communication opportunities at our institution. We have stationery designed for weekly inserts of special programs; maintain an Internet and Intranet presence; post articles and announcements in the institution's weekly *FYI* patient newsletter; faculty and staff newsletters; present information on M. D. Anderson's internal TV channel; and include information in the new patient information packets and guides for community physicians. We staff exhibits for cancer populations and healthcare professionals at conferences and workshops both on campus in the community and nationally and routinely provide in-services and make presentations to departments and clinics throughout the institution as well as to community agencies. M. D. Anderson's Department of Communications also coordinates media opportunities from local TV to national radio. It is important to investigate the educational forums that are already in place and contact the coordinators to secure an education session on CIM.

5.5 Research

Our research focuses on intervention programs to reduce the negative effects of cancer diagnosis and treatment and improve treatment outcomes and quality of life. Many patients, under the careful guidance of their physicians, are involved in research about mind-body medicine, acupuncture, dietary supplements and other regimens, and biopharmacologic agents such as vitamins and herbal preparations and other biologically based products. In fact, there is ongoing research in all CIM domains (mind-body medicine, energy based therapies, body-manipulative systems, alternative medical systems, and biologically based approaches). Below we list a few examples of the ongoing research (for details on the mind-body research see Chapter 10). For example, we are

- Studying the bio-behavioral effects of mind/body-based interventions such as stress management, including Indian-based Yoga, Tibetan-based Yoga, Qigong, meditation, music therapy, expressive writing, and other behavioral approaches.
- Examining the anticancer potential of natural animal or plant compounds such as dietary supplements, vitamins, and herbal remedies. Products being studied include green tea, turmeric, oleander, melatonin, shark cartilage, fish oil, mushrooms, and many others.
- Using acupuncture to treat some common cancer treatment-related side effects, including prolonged postoperative ileus, xerostomia, nausea, and others. Determining the biological bases of acupuncture also is an important part of this research endeavor.
- Examining traditional Chinese medicine for cancer. Part of this research is being done with colleagues at the Fudan University Cancer Hospital in Shanghai, China. The purpose of this research is to study three main areas of traditional Chinese medicine: natural products research, acupuncture research, and the mind/body practice of Qigong.
- Examining ways of utilizing qualitative research methods as part of mixed-method research methodology to evaluate patient perspectives on issues related to cancer care and CIM use.

5.6 Summary

Collaboration remains the key to the evolving clinical, educational, and research efforts of the Integrative Medicine Program. Our program has significantly increased awareness about CIM and its use by allopathic medical professionals dealing with cancer throughout the United States and the world. In this chapter, we have described how to establish an integrative medicine program from the clinical side of the screening of participants to the credentialing of providers to adhering to institutional policies and procedures and developing important educational forums for education faculty and staff. These collaborative processes are important because they encourage alliances to be formed with key stakeholders and parts of the institution necessary to implement and evaluate programs. These groups will be partners for years to come. Joining forces with those who can provide education in a variety of formats has been critical to developing Web tools to support patients, families, faculty, and staff in making decisions about CIM use. In implementing the Integrative Medicine Program at M. D. Anderson over the past several years, we recognized the increasing use of CIM and have responded accordingly.

For more information visit our Web site at www.mdanderson.org/departments/intmedprogram or call 713-794-4700.

Acknowledgments We thank Dr. Moshe Frenkel for his helpful and insightful input on this chapter.

References

1. Eisenberger DM, Davies RB, Ettner SL. Trends in alternative medicine use in the United States, 1990–1997: results of a follow-up national survey. JAMA 1998;280:1569–75.
2. Tasaki K, Maskarinec G, Shumay DM, Tatsumura Y, Kakai H. Communication between physicians and cancer patients about complementary and alternative medicine: exploring patients' perspectives. [see comment]. Psychooncology 2002;11(3):212–20.
3. Navo MA, Phan J, Vaughan C, Palmer JL, Michaud L, Jones KL, et al. An assessment of the utilization of complementary and alternative medication in women with gynecologic or breast malignancies. J Clin Oncol 2004;22(4):671–7.
4. Richardson MA, Sanders T, Palmer JL, Greisinger A, Singletary SE. Complementary/alternative medicine use in a comprehensive cancer center and the implications for oncology. J Clin Oncol 2000;18(13):2505–14.
5. Deng G, Cassileth BR, Yeung KS. Complementary therapies for cancer-related symptoms. J Support Oncol 2004;2(5):419–26.

Chapter 6
The Integrative Medicine Service at Memorial Sloan-Kettering Cancer Center

Barrie Cassileth and Jyothirmai Gubili

Contents

6.1	Introduction	67
6.2	Clinical Services	70
6.3	Therapies Offered and Related Research	72
6.4	Summary	78
References		78

Abstract Many cancer patients experience painful physical and emotional symptoms associated with cancer and cancer treatments. Integrative medicine combines mainstream cancer treatments and evidence-based complementary modalities such as touch therapies, music therapy, meditation, yoga, and acupuncture to provide symptom relief and to improve quality of life. The Integrative Medicine Service is an important component of Memorial Sloan-Kettering Cancer Center and has established complementary medicine as a valued element in cancer care.

Keywords: Cancer · symptom control · complementary therapies · integrative oncology.

6.1 Introduction

Modern diagnostic and therapeutic techniques have led to a dramatic increase in survival rates following completion of cancer treatment. In the United States, five-year survival rates across all cancer diagnoses approach 65% as of this writing. Today's diagnostic and therapeutic technologies lie behind these statistics, and they have eventuated in the 10 million U.S. citizens alive today 5 years after treatment for cancer.

J. Gubili
Memorial Sloan-Kettering Cancer Center, 1429 First Avenue, New York, NY 10021
e-mail: gubilij@mskcc.org

L. Cohen, M. Markman (eds.), *Integrative Oncology: Incorporating Complementary Medicine into Conventional Cancer Care*, © 2008 Humana Press, Totowa, NJ

These effective interventions, however, come at a cost. They are difficult and associated with short- and long-term toxicities. These troubling physical and emotional symptoms include hot flashes, xerostomia or extreme dry mouth, muscle atrophy, sensory dysfunction, peripheral neuropathy, pain, anxiety, and many other problems.

Many of these symptoms, while not always well managed by pharmaceuticals and other mainstream means, are nonetheless responsive to the pre-scientific techniques with which early cultures attempted to heal illnesses. These ancient approaches include touch therapies, music therapy, meditation, yoga, acupuncture, and more. Botanicals also may play a role. Contrary to single-molecule agents, such as chemotherapy and other prescription pharmaceuticals, botanical agents are collections of constituents that work synergistically. Less powerful but more gentle than prescription drugs, they may prove to play several roles such as enhancing immune function, reducing inflammation, and calming distress.

Both modern technology (to sustain and improve cure rates) and complementary therapies (to manage symptoms) are needed for today's cancer care. Together these approaches produce Integrative Oncology, a synthesis of the best of mainstream cancer treatment and evidence-based complementary therapies.

6.1.1 Emergence of the MSKCC Integrative Medicine Service

In 1999, the Board and leadership of Memorial Sloan-Kettering Cancer Center (MSKCC) completed many months of discussion about developing an "Integrative Medicine" entity, as it was termed, a program that would help patients through the vicissitudes of cancer treatment and beyond. The concept was to complement the outstanding cancer care provided at MSKCC by addressing everything but the tumor. That is, addressing cancer's emotional, physical, and spiritual side effects.

This was to realize the dream of Laurance S. Rockefeller, then Chairman of the MSKCC Board of Advisors and long-time supporter of cancer research and attention to patient and family needs. It was he who insisted that "Bodymindspirit" be inscribed on the wall of the main MSKCC outpatient Pavilion where others had wanted his name to appear. It was the author's great honor and joy to have known this uniquely humble and brilliant visionary and to bring his dream to life.

The author was asked to join the MSKCC faculty and to design and implement an Integrative Medicine Service (Fig. 6.1). She soon presented the MSKCC Board and leadership with the organizational plan outlined below. This plan was based on creating a department consistent with that seen in any academic medicine setting. It included the three basic components of departments in medical centers: inpatient and outpatient care, research, and education. It was standard in terms of organization, but not in terms of how it fit into the accepted conceptual framework of most analogous settings. This would be a horizontal entity, and it would provide a set of programs previously unavailable at MSKCC and not available elsewhere in its breadth and depth. It would also include a web-based information service. This

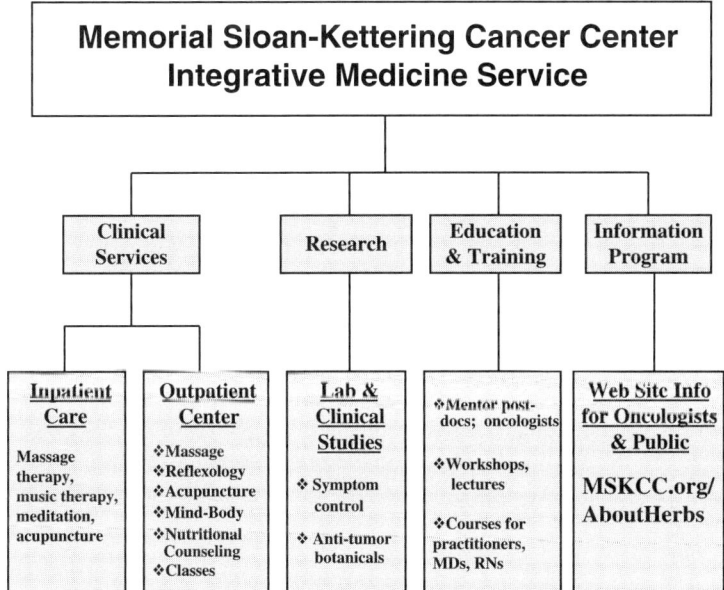

Fig. 6.1 The Integrative Medicine Service at Memorial Sloan-Kettering Cancer Center

department was specifically designed to serve as a prototype so that others could learn from it and use relevant components, altered as needed to fit institutional and geographic cultures elsewhere.

6.1.2 Role of Integrative Medicine at MSKCC

The "Integrative Medicine Service" was so titled by the MSKCC Board and leadership. The "Service" designation, as well as backing from those at the highest institutional levels, afforded a respectability and profile that enabled this new entity to grow and become a success. Cardiology is also a "service" at MSKCC. Clearly, the term "Service" is applied to major, often horizontal departments that serve the MSKCC community. Integrative Medicine was created as a horizontal program, cutting across the cancer-specific departments and ready to work with all groups equally.

Today, 7 years hence, clinicians, researchers, and staff throughout the institution collaborate regularly on Integrative Medicine's basic science and clinical projects. Like all academic medicine departments, the Integrative Medicine Service cares for inpatients and outpatients, conducts research, and provides training for medical staff, students, and the public. It also reaches out to the local community by providing outpatient services and programs for all patients. As of this writing, the Service has over 1000 patient visits each month, a substantial roster of funded laboratory and clinical research projects, a very active educational web site and many training programs.

The center clearly distinguishes between complementary and alternative therapies. This distinction is important in terms of clinical efficacy so that the MSKCC as well as the outside community clearly understands the perspective of the Service Chief and the basic principles on which the Integrative Medicine Service was built. Our standards are high and identical to those of MSKCC, as we too hold ourselves to a rigorous scientific approach. Unproven or disproved "alternative therapies" are falsely promoted as viable cancer treatments and sometimes as cancer cures and often sold for use instead of mainstream therapy. Complementary therapies, in contrast, are used as adjuncts to needed mainstream care for the management of symptoms and to enhance well-being. Complementary therapies address body, mind, and spirit, aiming to control pain and other symptoms and to optimize quality of life for patients and families. This definition is very similar to the World Health Organization's definition of palliative care. The Integrative Medicine program serves as the quality of life arm of cancer care at MSKCC.

6.2 Clinical Services

The Integrative Medicine Service treats both inpatients and outpatients. Clinical services are geared to manage both physical and emotional symptoms that patients experience. Patients who are hospitalized can either self-refer or may be referred by MSKCC physicians or other health professionals. Requests for inpatient services are handled by an Integrative Medicine staff person via a phone line designated for this purpose. Inpatient requests are reviewed and prioritized. Patients in critical need and those who are terminally ill are given top priority and seen within 12–24 h. Other requests are handled as soon as possible, usually within 24–48 h and as therapist time permits. Among requests from inpatient floors, massage therapy and music therapy predominate, although acupuncture, mind-body therapies, and in-bed yoga are also provided. All inpatient services are provided at no charge to patients.

Outpatient services are available at the Bendheim Integrative Medicine Center, a free-standing building located six blocks from the main MSKCC hospital. This space was designed to provide a soothing, non-biomedical atmosphere that in and of itself contributes to patients' feelings of security and well-being. A large, open lobby (Fig. 6.2) contains vaulted windows, a flowing water sculpture, art, many plants, and comfortable chairs arranged in small groupings.

A group exercise room with mirrored walls and hard wood floor provides space for yoga, aerobics, and many classes, such as chair aerobics and Qi Gong.

6 Integrative Medicine Service

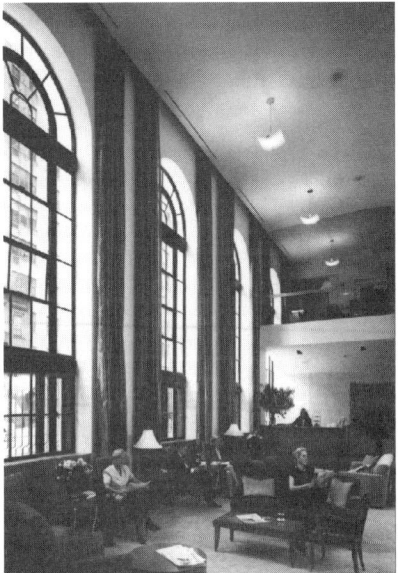

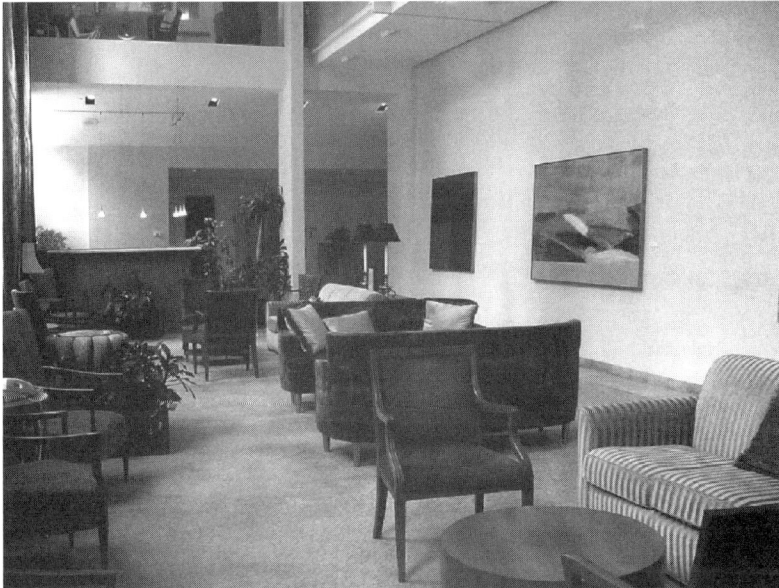

Fig. 6.2 Integrative Medicine Center Lobby

A room with natural light streaming from a large skylight, comfortable reclining chairs, provides soothing space for individual or small group sessions of meditation, guided imagery, hypnosis, and other mind-body therapies for patients and family members. There is also ample office space elsewhere in the building for the administrative and research aspects of the program, as well as a large conference room and offices for managers of the primary clinical programs.

Outpatient therapies at the Bendheim Integrative Medicine Center are available to MSKCC patients and family members and also to faculty and staff, patients from other hospitals, and members of the community. All outpatient sessions and classes are provided on an appointment, fee-for-service basis.

6.3 Therapies Offered and Related Research

Starting initially with massage therapies and music therapy, the menu of services quickly expanded to include acupuncture, meditation, relaxation and other mind-body therapies, fitness and nutrition, and numerous classes plus lectures for patients and the community. Some therapies, including music, dance, and fitness programs, were modified for MSKCC's large pediatric population and have become an important part of the care of children with cancer in our institution.

6.3.1 Touch Therapy

There are multiple methodologies for touching the skin and manipulating muscles and soft tissue to provide comfort. Swedish massage, most commonly used in North America, involves six basic strokes—effleurage, petrissage, friction, tapotement, compression, and vibration (Fig. 6.3). Swedish massage is thought to improve circulation and relax muscles. Shiatsu, a massage technique developed in Japan, involves pressure to acupoints to relieve tension. For reflexology, specific points on the feet,

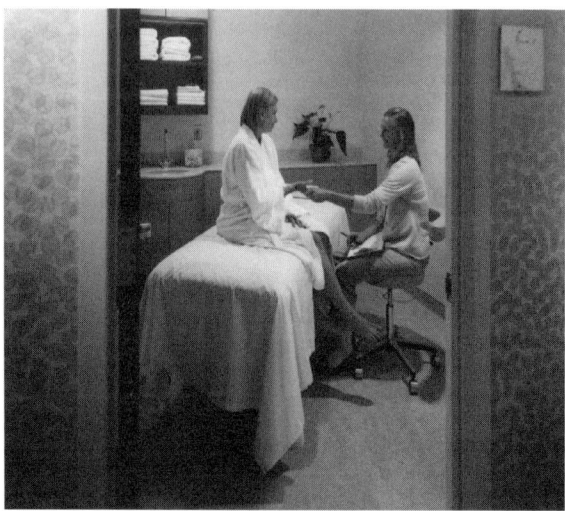

Fig. 6.3 Integrative Medicine Center massage therapy room

hands, and ears are pressed to reduce stress, relieve pain, and enhance well-being. Reiki is a type of light-touch massage; the practitioner lays hands on a fully clothed patient who is relaxing on a massage table. This light-touch method has been especially useful in working with end-stage cancer patients. Thai massage is a form of touch therapy that has been used for centuries to relieve muscle tension, increase flexibility, and promote overall relaxation.

For cancer patients to receive maximum benefit from massage, therapists vary pressure and duration of body work according to the patient's clinical status. Massage therapists at MSKCC are licensed, experienced practitioners who then received special training in working with cancer patients.

The Integrative Medicine Service conducted a large study of massage for cancer patients. This study was done over a period of 3 years and involved 1290 patients. Massage, light touch massage, and foot massage were administered to patients. Patients rated the severity of symptoms including pain, fatigue, stress, nausea, and depression pre and post-massage therapy. Data indicate that symptom scores were reduced by 50% with outpatients improving 10% more than inpatients. In addition, follow-up showed that the benefits of massage persisted for 48 h [1]. These results led to a randomized trial, currently underway, to evaluate the benefits of massage for pain management in cancer patients for longer periods of time.

6.3.2 Music Therapy

Music has been a part of the human experience since ancient times, marking important private and communal events and serving as a centerpiece for daily activities. Music affects people deeply and has the capacity to sooth, energize, or call to action. Every culture has its music, which often originated in efforts to mimic sounds found in nature using simple pipes, drums, and strings. The use of music for healing and spiritual ceremonies predates the written word and may even predate language. The benefits of music therapy, which involves a trained practitioner who uses music to reach therapeutic goals, include a period free from interruption, the companionship and skills of the therapist, and live, soothing music.

Formalized music therapy, the use of music by a trained practitioner on a patient, has been studied for close to 70 years. In 1944, Michigan State University offered the first degree-awarding program in music therapy, establishing the field as a healthcare profession. Today, over 5000 professional music therapists work in the U.S. health care system [2].

The MSKCC Integrative medicine Service conducted a randomized, controlled clinical trial to assess the ability of music therapy to reduce mood disturbance in patients awaiting autologous stem cell transplantation for hematologic malignancies. This procedure causes significant psychological distress. Sixty-nine patients awaiting transplantation participated in this study. Patients were randomized to music therapy given by trained music therapists versus standard care. Results showed that anxiety and depression scores were significantly reduced in patients receiving music therapy compared to those in the control (usual care) group [3].

6.3.3 Acupuncture

Acupuncture, a treatment modality used initially in traditional Chinese medicine and increasingly accepted today in the West, involves the stimulation of one or more predetermined points on the body with needles, heat, pressure, or electricity for therapeutic effect. It is based on the ancient theory of balance between yin and yang and the flow of Qi (energy) along hypothesized vertical channels, or "meridians," in the body. Acupuncture points are located at specific locations along the channels. The flow of Qi, and therefore, health, was thought to be regulated by needling these points.

Traditionally trained acupuncturists examine the tongue and palpate the pulse to assess the patient's condition, while Western trained medical practitioners usually perform standard physical examinations. Following determination of a treatment plan for problems identified, needles are inserted into relevant acupuncture points and retained for 20–30 min. Acupuncture points usually are located in depressions between joints, muscle fascia, or sensitive points along hypothesized channels.

The anatomic structures representing meridians have not been identified to date. However, some acupuncture points coincide with trigger points that are sensitive to pressure, indicating enriched enervation at the anatomic location. Electroacupuncture, moxibustion, and acupressure are also used in addition to needling for increased stimulation.

Cancer patients seek acupuncture for chemotherapy-induced nausea and vomiting, fatigue, hot flashes, neuropathy, and pain. Acupuncturists use a combination of standard needling and electrostimulation as appropriate for each individual patient.

The Integrative Medicine Service team of acupuncturists and researchers has collaborated in the conduct of multiple clinical trials on acupuncture for the relief of various side effects. We conducted a prospective randomized trial to determine whether acupuncture reduces post-chemotherapy fatigue. Thirty-one patients who had completed chemotherapy but experienced persisting fatigue were enrolled in two cohorts. Patients received acupuncture either twice a week for 4 weeks or once a week for 6 weeks. The primary end point was change in score on the Brief Fatigue Inventory between baseline and 2 weeks after the final treatment. Results showed a 31.1% improvement following acupuncture with no important difference between once-weekly and twice-weekly treatments [4]. Based on these data, a randomized placebo-controlled trial is underway.

We also evaluated the benefits of acupuncture in the control of post-thoracotomy pain in a pilot trial. Thirty-six patients scheduled for unilateral thoracotomy were treated with acupuncture. Eighteen semi-permanent intradermal needles were inserted on either side of the spine. Needles were removed after 4 weeks. Pain was measured on the first 5 postoperative days and following discharge, at 7, 30, 60, and 90 days. The treatment was not only well tolerated by 75% patients but there were also no reports of adverse events. The data also showed decreasing severity of pain over time [5].

A phase III trial is currently underway to assess the effects of acupuncture for the treatment of pain and dysfunction commonly experienced following neck dissection. Research is also being conducted to determine the neurologic changes caused by acupuncture in healthy patients using fMRI technology. Saliva production is monitored during this study as well in hopes of finding the best acupuncture approach to improve saliva production in patients whose salivary glands were damaged by radiation therapy.

6.3.4 Mind-Body Therapies

Meditation, mindfulness based stress reduction, guided imagery, self-hypnosis, and pre-surgery self-hypnosis have been demonstrated effective for problems associated with cancer and cancer treatment. A licensed clinical psychologist manages the Integrative Medicine Mind-Body Program. She trains individual patients to focus on the present by concentrating on breathing and works with those anticipating surgery to use self-hypnosis to induce a state of calm that typically facilitates physical and emotional response to surgery. These one-on-one sessions are offered bedside to inpatients, or at the Bendheim Integrative Medicine Center meditation room for outpatients, in one-on-one or small group sessions as needed prior to surgery. Additionally, a group of meditators attend the weekly Advanced Mindfulness Practice Group.

6.3.5 Movement/Fitness Program

The fitness needs of the MSKCC cancer patients are met through multiple classes offered to outpatients, community, and staff at the Integrative Medicine Center. A wide variety of classes are offered including "Strong Bones," focused fitness for women, chair aerobics, pilates, and combinations of mind-body and music therapies. Many classes have been developed for cancer patients such as light workout, an exercise program specially designed for those who have completed cancer treatment, which combines weight training, stretching, and dance to increase muscle strength, flexibility, balance, and endurance. A pilot study is planned to determine the ability of exercise to improve disease-free survival following a diagnosis of breast or colorectal cancer. Patients with early stage breast cancer undergoing surgery to remove the tumor will be randomized to exercise or control groups. Both aerobic and resistance training will be offered to those in the exercise group. We hope that this study will develop the research structure for a randomized trial.

Qi Gong, an ancient system of exercise comprising a series of gentle movements and meditation, helps reduce stress and improves stamina and sleep. Yoga promotes healing and relaxation. One of our Yoga therapists visits inpatients in their hospital rooms for one-on-one Yoga sessions taught at bedside. Movements are modified to meet the limitations imposed by the patient's clinical status, hospital equipment, and pain.

The Integrative Medicine Service also has a strong dance therapy program for pediatric patients. This is a method for using movement, sound, and motion—all the senses—to help babies and small children cope with painful procedures and treatments.

6.3.6 Nutrition

Many patients and family members seek nutritional counseling from the Integrative Medicine Service. Some clients are healthy community members looking for guidance on dietary regimes. Others seek a diet to help them prolong their state of health after discovering that they are carrying a gene that makes them prone to a disease. The majority of patients seen are referrals from the main cancer hospital. In addition to the registered dietitians available to patients at the main campus of MSKCC, the Integrative Medicine Service employs a RD with specific training on the proper use of supplements for disease prevention. This background allows him to provide scientifically based recommendations for healthy eating and to encourage optimal well-being for patients about to begin or in treatment for cancer.

Integrative Medicine's dietitian validates truly helpful dietary changes and explains the myths and dangers of radical diets. He offers phone and office consultations and teaches small evening classes for patients and their families. In the class, patients are introduced to what diet has to offer for symptom relief and disease prevention. During individual consultations, the dietitian makes recommendations specific to the patient, disease, and point in time. Dietary recommendations for the same patient may vary with course of disease, for example, a patient may need one diet for controlling symptoms of chemotherapy and another diet if a secondary cancer is found. This customization of diet helps relieve patients of the stress of shifting through the plethora of information available on cancer and diet.

Our nutritional counseling program also addresses the many issues of concern to patients about herbs and other botanicals. Our AboutHerbs website also provides helpful information to patients and family members about herb–drug interactions and explains why most herbs should be avoided during receipt of chemotherapy, radiation therapy, or pending surgery.

6.3.7 Immune-Modulating Botanicals Research

In addition to ongoing studies to investigate the role of acupuncture, massage, music therapy, mind-body therapies, exercise/fitness, and other complementary therapies to control the side effects of cancer treatment, the Integrative Medicine Service also maintains a major interest in studying botanicals for their potential effectiveness as anti-cancer agents. Some botanicals may have important benefits against cancer.

Our NIH-designated Botanicals Research Center, the "Memorial Sloan-Kettering Research Center for Botanical Immunomodulators," supports our collaboration with the Institute of Chinese Medicine in Hong Kong, two laboratories at MSKCC, and one each at Cornell-Weill and Rockefeller Universities, systematically investigates immune-modulating botanical supplements, their composition, and mechanisms of action. It was founded in May 2005 to investigate immune-modulating botanicals, bringing best results to clinical trails. This is one of six NIH-supported botanical research centers in the United States. The clinical implications of the Center's work are comprehensive, including cancer prevention and treatment, management of treatment complications, heath maintenance, and survivorship.

6.3.8 Education and Training

The Integrative Medicine Service educates patients, caregivers, and medical professionals about the many aspects of complementary medicine. Our "Integrative Oncology Fellowship Training program," the first such to be awarded by the National Institutes of Health, will enable physicians to train for clinical and research careers using complementary therapies and botanicals.

For licensed massage therapists and acupuncturists, the center offers specialized classes in working with cancer patients. In the 4 years since "Medical Massage for the Cancer Patient" was first offered, we have trained more than 500 massage therapists from North America and elsewhere. This course prepares experienced practitioners to determine a clinically based treatment plan for each patient, to safely and effectively provide therapeutic touch, and to meet the challenges and reap the rewards of working in a cancer patient practice.

Similarly, our two and one-half day "Acupuncture for the Cancer Patient" course prepares certified, experienced acupuncturists to work with cancer patients. Both sets of courses offer basic and advanced training in the common cancers such as breast, colorectal, lung, and prostate, their management and clinical course, and detail how massage or acupuncture for cancer patients differs from that of general practice. Patient assessment and treatment appropriate to various levels of patient clinical status is provided, as is the management of difficult situations, special clinical issues, legal issue, and so on.

Our Music Therapy Program offers accredited student internships for graduate and undergraduate students in music therapy. Topics include how music therapy in palliative care differs from that with other groups, the psychosocial and spiritual needs and coping styles of patients and families, patient assessment and goal development, and music therapy techniques for pediatric and adult patients.

6.3.9 Information Program: AboutHerbs Web site (www.mskcc.org/aboutherbs)

Cancer patients are more likely than the general public to use dietary supplements, sometimes in hopes of improving chances for cancer cure, and often to relieve the symptoms associated with cancer treatments. The potential for adverse effects and interactions with anticancer drugs is a major concern. Because the availability of reliable, frequently updated information on dietary supplements is limited, the Integrative Medicine Service maintains a free Web site, "AboutHerbs." Launched in November 2002, this site provides objective information on herbs, vitamins, dietary supplements, and unproved cancer therapies. The site serves both healthcare professionals and the public. It was named one of the top five web sites in all of Medicine by Scientific American in 2003 and continues to be mentioned in news, magazines, and online publications. The web site has registered more than 4 million hits since its inception and currently contains 217 monographs. Each monograph includes a clinical summary and details about constituents, adverse effects, interactions, and potential benefits or adverse effects.

AboutHerbs is supported by a dedicated editorial team and an Advisory Board of experts in Integrative Medicine, oncology, nutrition, pharmacy, and patient advocacy. Information on the site is updated frequently to reflect the latest knowledge and scientific evidence.

6.4 Summary

Seven years after its creation, the Integrative Medicine Service today is a well-established, integral feature of the MSKCC with 60 full- and part-time therapists, research staff, AboutHerbs managers, and administrative personnel. This team combines its skills to offer a full package of services to inpatients, outpatients, staff, and the larger community and to conduct rigorous research at bench and bedside. The knowledge gained from these and other evidence-based approaches is shared with patients, caregivers, and the community through a web site, informational pamphlets, talks, and lectures. Formal classes and training sessions further establish complementary medicine as an important element in cancer care.

References

1. Cassileth BR, Vickers AJ. Massage therapy for symptom control: outcome study at a major cancer center. *J Pain Symptom Manage* 2004;28(3):244–9.
2. Cassileth BR, Deng G, Vickers AJ, et al. *PDQ Integrative Oncology: Complementary Therapies in Cancer Care.* 2005, Hamilton, Ontario: BC Decker Inc.
3. Cassileth BR, Vickers AJ, Magill LA. Music therapy for mood disturbance during hospitalization for autologous stem cell transplantation: a randomized controlled trial. *Cancer* 2003;98(12):2723–9.
4. Vickers AJ, Straus DJ, Fearon B, et al. Acupuncture for postchemotherapy fatigue: a phase II study. *J Clin Oncol* 2004;22(9):1731–5.
5. Vickers AJ, Rusch VW, Malhotra VT, et al. Acupuncture is a feasible treatment for post-thoracotomy pain: results of a prospective pilot trial. *BMC Anesthesiol* 2006;6:5.

Chapter 7
Integrative Oncology—Leonard P. Zakim Center

The Dana-Farber Cancer Institute Experience

David S. Rosenthal, Anne Doherty-Gilman, Cynthia Medeiros, Susan DeCristofaro, and Elizabeth Dean-Clower

Contents

7.1	Introduction	80
7.2	Mission Statement	81
7.3	Policies and Procedures	83
7.4	Documentation and Scheduling of Integrative Therapies	89
7.5	Zakim Center Collaborations	92
7.6	Growth of the Zakim Center	93
7.7	Financials	95
7.8	Creating an Integrative Education Program for Patients and Families, Physicians, Nurses, and Researchers	97
7.9	Development of a Research Program	100
7.10	Concluding Thoughts	102
	References	103

Abstract More and more frequently, hospitals are expanding their services to incorporate complementary therapies into their medical settings. One of the first successful models for a hospital-based integrative therapies center was developed in Boston, Massachusetts at Dana-Farber Cancer Institute, a Harvard University academic medical center and world-renowned cancer patient care and research institute. Driven by patient advocacy and a desire to provide the most safe and efficacious care possible, the Leonard P. Zakim Center for Integrative Therapies at Dana-Farber unites leading cancer experts with complementary therapy practitioners in order to offer patients a more holistic, comprehensive cancer care. The Zakim Center is an interdisciplinary program that uses a three-prong approach by offering

---

D. Rosenthal
Director, Harvard University Health Service, Co-Director, Zakim Center for Integrative Therapies, Dana-Farber Cancer Institute, Professor of Medicine, Harvard Medical School, Henry K. Oliver Professor of Hygiene, Harvard University, 75 Mount Auburn St., Cambridge, MA 02138
e-mail: drose@uhs.harvard.edu

complementary therapies including acupuncture, massage, nutrition, and others to enhance patients' quality of life and to help them with symptom management, while at the same time, educating staff and patients about these therapies and researching them in order to advance their scientific evidence base. Development of this Center and the concept of a new discipline, "integrative oncology,' required much communication, strategic planning, leadership commitment, and the diligence of many individuals. Through focused program and operational development, active institutional collaborations, and the concerted efforts of the whole Dana-Farber community, a premier comprehensive integrative therapies center that is affordable and accessible was established and continues to flourish and grow extensively today to meet the needs of patients, clinicians, and researchers at Dana-Farber Cancer Institute.

Keywords: Integrative oncology · integrative therapies · cancer care · complementary therapies · program development · quality of life · patient empowerment · Zakim Center · integration strategies · acupuncture · massage therapy · Reiki · nutrition · integrative oncology consultation · Qigong · staffing model · documentation · Dana-Farber.

7.1 Introduction

7.1.1 Development of the Concept of Integrative Oncology at DFCI and First Steps

"It takes one person to start a revolution----"

The concept of an Integrative Therapies Center at Dana-Farber Cancer Institute (DFCI) began in 1995. Leonard P. (Lenny) Zakim, Executive Director of the New England region of the Anti-Defamation League and a patient with multiple myeloma, advocated for the establishment of a complementary therapies program for cancer patients at the Boston-based hospital. Mr. Zakim wrote, "For a patient seeking to play an active role in his/her treatment and to regain some measure of control, complementary therapies are valuable steps towards patient well-being and empowerment. My physician and I ultimately became partners in connecting the best treatments of the East and West for me."

Zakim's appeal as a leading member of Boston's political and civil rights communities helped spark quick interest. Friends and colleagues began to donate to a DFCI Complementary Therapies Fund, and a multidisciplinary committee was established to explore the development of such a program. This multidisciplinary Task Force, co-chaired by Zakim and the Director of Patient and Family Support Services, was charged by the Executive Management Committee of DFCI to:

1. explore the feasibility of establishing a complementary and alternative medicine (CAM) program at DFCI and
2. develop an educational video on the use of complementary therapies for cancer patients.

The committee included patients, family members, staff from every discipline within DFCI, trustees of the Institute, community CAM practitioners, and representatives from area hospitals. Four standing committees were created: Adult Clinical, Education, Research, and Pediatric. Each committee developed short- and long-term goals.

In January 1998, Dr. David Eisenberg, Director of the Harvard Medical School's Osher Institute, Division for Research and Education in Complementary and Integrative Medical Therapies, gave the first lecture on CAM to DFCI clinical and research staff.

In the fall of 1999, a video entitled "Complementary Therapies: Empowering the Cancer Patient," featuring DFCI patients, physicians, and complementary therapy providers was completed [1]. In October 1999, members of the task force formed "Team Lenny," a group of walkers who participated in the DFCI annual Jimmy Fund Walk (JFW) and raised over $8000 to further the work of developing the program. A Program Director, Medical Director, and Executive Director were appointed.

Despite being weakened by the final stages of his disease, Zakim spoke powerfully about CAM at a DFCI fundraising event late in 1999. The President of the Institute agreed to further fundraising and the "Friends of Lenny" Committee was formed. Their task was to raise $1 million in Zakim's honor. Although he died just a few months later in December 1999, Lenny was aware of the final plans. A year later, with $1 million raised, the ribbon was cut on the Leonard P. Zakim Center for Integrative Therapies.

As the Center grew, additional staff were brought on to provide administrative support. The Task Force was replaced by a formal Zakim Center Executive Committee, comprised of key Institute decision makers, DFCI physicians, nurses, social workers, and other clinicians from a variety of disciplines, and communications and development personnel, as well as cancer patients and family members. This group provided advice on policy, program development, operations, and strategic planning; one of its initial steps was to finalize a mission statement.

7.2 Mission Statement

> The Leonard P. Zakim Center for Integrative Therapies at Dana-Farber Cancer Institute is dedicated to enhancing the quality of life for cancer patients and families by incorporating complementary and alternative medicine into traditional cancer care. The center is committed to making services affordable and accessible to pediatric and adult patients and through clinical services and education seeks to empower patients to actively participate in their treatment plans. By conducting peer-reviewed, evidence-based research, the center will build knowledge about the effectiveness of these therapies.

7.2.1 Operational Development

In early fall 1999, before start-up funding was secured, a program manager with a background in integrative therapy program development, management, and research was hired to join DFCI and work with the Task Force. Although a passionate Task Force existed, it was made up of volunteers, with full-time jobs who could not focus fully on this major integration effort. The program manager was charged with the following:

1. managing the on-going efforts to integrate complementary therapies; and
2. serving as a liaison to groups at DFCI and in the community who were working on similar efforts.

When funding was secured, the goal was widened: to develop a clinical, educational, and research complementary therapies program at DFCI. Although some complementary therapy initiatives were underway at Dana-Farber, they were not happening in a cohesive, efficient manner. Several options were considered. Should the focus be on research and have that drive the clinical program? Should efforts be put into education and have that be the vehicle for integration? Should a formal clinical program be offered with an expertise that DFCI clinicians could come to rely on? Or, should each of these areas be developed simultaneously? Leadership decided upon the latter.

Another avenue that was considered to help support the center's work was clinical research. Research possibilities were evaluated, and the practitioners were committed to conducting evidence-based studies to promote integrative medicine. It was the firm belief that applying the stringent standards of conventional clinical research to the analysis of CAM therapies would help to demystify them while at the same time determine which interventions worked. This approach would also be consistent with the DFCI mission of "advancing cancer care through research" (see Section 8.2).

Networking with other cancer national centers and the Greater Boston community helped benchmark and set program goals. A new video, *Complementary Therapies: Empowering the Cancer Patient*, was mailed to all major cancer centers and programs in the United States, helped to open a dialogue with colleagues nationwide.

Organizationally, the Zakim program was first housed within Dana-Farber's department of Patient and Family Support Services, which resided in the Department of Nursing and Patient Care Services. It was important that integrative therapies be truly integrated into the fabric of the Institute. To accomplish this goal, clinical space and administrative offices needed to be found. The pros and cons of an on-site versus off-site program were weighed. With space off-site, there would be more room, more services, and more accessibility. Holding the program on-site, however, would give us the ability to be truly integrated into DFCI, allowed integrative therapy providers to interact with physicians and nurses, write in the same electronic medical record (EMR), and share the same workrooms. This was the direction we decided to pursue. A newly renovated and yet-to-be-assigned DFCI building opened in the spring of 2000, and successful advocacy placed the Zakim Center's administrative offices in a prominent location therein: an administrative suite of three offices occupying one-half of the first floor lobby. The space was centrally located in an area where patients and clinicians frequent.

The integrative therapy program was now, physically, on the map at DFCI. But while administrative space had been secured, the need still existed for clinical treatment space and a decision on which therapies to offer. Staff pondered the possibilities. What therapies were patients most frequently using in the community? Which therapies showed the most promise for helping cancer patients? Which could be easily integrated into a hospital setting? It was discovered that a nurse practitioner trained in mind-body therapy techniques offered guided imagery and therapeutic touch on a part-time basis in Dana-Farber's infusion areas and exam rooms. After discussion, a policy statement on complementary therapy use at DFCI was created: "After careful study and consideration of our community and institutional needs, DFCI has chosen to incorporate complementary therapies into the services we offer. Initially, we are limiting the complementary services offered to massage therapy, acupuncture, Reiki, mind body therapies, and nutritional counseling."

Several staffing models were discussed. They are the following:

1. Contracting with another department to offer services;
2. Hiring practitioners directly into the Zakim Center as staff members of DFCI;
3. Incorporating the use of volunteers; and/or
4. Bringing providers on as consultants.

Over time, each of these arrangements was used.

In the beginning, approval was obtained to hire several providers on a part-time basis: an acupuncturist for one 4-h session per week, a massage therapist for 20 h per week, and a nutritionist who would focus on holistic nutrition for 20 h per week. The acupuncturist and massage therapist were hired directly into the Zakim Center and the nutritionist hired into the Department of Nutrition. In addition, two nurses already on staff at DFCI who practiced Reiki outside the Institute were assigned designated time by their departments to provide Reiki during their regular nursing work schedule.

7.3 Policies and Procedures

Having identified the services to offer, the next step for the Zakim Center staff was developing credentialing criteria and privileging guidelines for CAM practitioners at DFCI. Working with the Institute's Medical Staff Executive Committee and Risk Management Department, the center drafted its first policies: Acupuncture Clinical Practice (Table 7.1) and Acupuncture Credentialing (Table 7.2). These policies addressed educational and experience requirements, references, and practice guidelines for acupuncture. Similar policies were developed for all complementary therapies, a process that took hours of research and discussion, as there was no clear consensus even within the CAM professions about what the necessary criteria should be for practitioners working in a hospital setting. In Massachusetts, for instance, acupuncturists are licensed by the Massachusetts Board of Registration in Medicine. Although Reiki itself is not licensed by the state, licensed RNs are able

Table 7.1 Dana-Farber Cancer Institute Acupuncture Policy

PURPOSE: To provide Acupuncture for pediatric and adult patients in the clinical areas.

SCOPE: This policy applies to all staff Acupuncturists employed by DFCI involved in the delivery of acupuncture care.

OBJECTIVES:

1. To promote relaxation and a sense of comfort.
2. To rebalance the Qi in order to support the immune system.
3. To alter the perception of pain, therefore alleviating discomfort.
4. To decrease anxiety and depression.

PROCEDURE: To provide safe and effective Traditional Chinese Medicine, specifically, acupuncture, for adult and pediatric patients. Acupuncturists shall practice strictly within the parameters of standard acupuncture training providing proof of graduation from an accredited school of Acupuncture.

Must be licensed to practice acupuncture in The Commonwealth of Massachusetts. Must maintain continuing education credits as required by the Committee on Acupuncture under the Board of Registration in Medicine in Massachusetts.

Procedures:

1. Review patient medical history and current health status.
2. Explain the procedure and discuss individualized treatment.
3. Limited physical exam: pulse taking and tongue observation.
4. Patient is placed in supportive position with appropriate areas exposed for treatment.
5. Acupuncturist puts on exam gloves.
6. Skin is prepared in sterile fashion with alcohol wipe.
7. Disposable sterile needles are placed at the acupuncture points chosen for each individual.
8. Needles are left in place for 10–30 minutes.
9. Patient is periodically checked for comfort and relaxation. Patient can notify acupuncturist by ringing bell if any discomfort occurs.
10. Needles are removed, further points may be chosen depending on individual's problem and response.
11. Used sharps are disposed in needle box.
12. Hands should be disinfected with a waterless hand agent before and after patient contact. Soap and water should be used only when hands are visibly soiled.
13. Documentation of the session and patients response, reassessment and follow-up plan.
14. Acupuncturists are under the supervision of the Medical Director or his designee of the Zakim Center.

References:

Board of Registration in Medicine, Committee on Acupuncture, Commonwealth of Massachusetts. The Massachusetts Regulations Governing the Practice of Acupuncture 243 CMR 5.00.

Cassidy, C, Chinese medicine users in the United States part II: preferred aspects of care, The Journal of Alternative and Complementary Medicine, Vol. 4, Number 2, 1998, 189–202.

Kemper KJ, Sarah R, Highfield ES, Xiaros E, Barnes L, Berde C, On pins and needles, pediatric patients[1] experience with acupuncture, Pediatrics 2000, Vol. 105, Number 4, 941–947.

Kemper KJ, Wornham WL, Consultations for holistic pediatric services for inpatient and outpatient oncology patients at a children's hospital. Arch Pediatric Adol Med. April 2001, Vol. 155, 449–454.

Table 7.1 (continued)

Moffet, H, Acupuncture and Oriental medicine update, Alternative & Complementary Therapies; July/August 1996.

National Institutes of Health, Consensus Development Conference Statement, November 3-5 1997.

Pomeranz B, Scientific Research into acupuncture for the relief of pain, Journal of Alternative and Complementary Medicine, Vol. 2, Number. 1, 1996, 53–60.

Yamashita H, Tsukayama H, Hori N, Kimura T, Yasuo Tanno. Incidence of adverse reactions associated with acupuncture. Journal of Alternative and Complementary Medicine, Vol. 6, Number. 4, 2000, 345–350.

Approved By: Zakim Center Executive Committee

Date: February 2002

Rev.: Zakim Center Executive Committee

Date: March 2005

Table 7.2 Dana-Farber Cancer Institute Medical Staff Policy

ACUPUNCTURE CREDENTIALING POLICY

POLICY:
It shall be the policy of the Dana-Farber Cancer Institute to initiate a sufficient screening process for credentialing Non-Physician Acupuncturists and Physician Acupuncturists to assure that only fully qualified practitioners provide medical care to Dana-Farber patients. Acupuncture may be performed only by a fully licensed physician who is a member of the DFCI Medical Staff or by an acupuncturist duly licensed by the Commonwealth of Massachusetts and whom a member of the DFCI Medical Staff supervises. These practitioners shall provide supporting documentation of his or her education, training and experience. All non-physician acupuncturists shall be hired through the Department of Human Resources in conjunction with the Leonard P. Zakim Center for Integrated Therapies.

DEFINITION:
Acupuncture is the practice of medicine based on traditional oriental medical theories, and involves (but is not limited to) the insertion of needles through the skin at certain points in the body, with or without the application of electric current, heat, or the topical use of herbs to relieve pain or improve bodily function. Electroacupuncture, whether utilizing electrodes on the surface of the skin or current applied to inserted needles and laser acupuncture are considered the practice of acupuncture.

PROCEDURE:
A. No individual may practice acupuncture at the Dana-Farber Cancer Institute until his/her credentials and qualifications have been reviewed and approved by the Medical Director of the Leonard P. Zakim Center for Integrated Therapies (DFCI) or his designee as described below. Only physician Acupuncturists will be required to go through the Dana-Farber Medical Staff Committee approval process. Non-Physician Acupuncturists must be credentialed according to the following criteria.

B. Criteria

1. For non-physicians, the individual must:

    a. Provide a copy of a valid and current Massachusetts license to practice acupuncture;
    b. provide a copy of the most recent completed application form for acupuncture licensure (Massachusetts);

Table 7.2 (continued)

    c. provide proof of malpractice insurance; and

    d. Provide three (3) letters of recommendation from persons knowledgeable in acupuncture and the individual's abilities, at least two (2) of which must be from individuals with current (within the past two years) knowledge of the applicant's abilities.

    e. Provide satisfactory evidence of at least thirty (30) accredited hours, over a three (3) year period, of continuing education in medical acupuncture.

    f. The individual must be reviewed and approved by the Medical Director of the Leonard P. Zakim Center for Integrated Therapies or his designee.

2. For physicians, the individual must:

    a. Be a member of the DFCI medical staff with current privileges and licensure. Requests for Acupuncture privileges must be independently reviewed in accordance with DFCI credentialing procedures.

    b. Have successfully completed at least two hundred (200) hours of graduate training in medical acupuncture of AMA category I certified programs or equivalents thereof, as determined by the American Academy of Medical Acupuncture;

    c. Provide three (3) letters of recommendation specifically addressing the individual's abilities and experience in acupuncture. At least one (1) of the letters must be from a teacher or supervisor, and at least two (2) of the letters must be from individuals with current (within the past two years) knowledge of the applicant's abilities; and

    d. Provide satisfactory evidence of at least thirty (30) accredited hours, over a three (3) year period, of continuing education in medical acupuncture.

    e. Renewal of medical staff privileges shall include a review of the individual's clinical experience and/or quality assurance data with regard to the practice of acupuncture.

SUPERVISION OF NON-PHYSICIAN ACUPUNCTURISTS

The Medical Director of the Leonard P. Zakim Center for Integrated Therapies or his designee shall be designated as the supervisor of all non-physician acupuncturists. The Director is not required to be physically present during the provision of acupuncture services by non-physician acupuncturists.

The Director's supervisory responsibilities shall include confirmation of compliance with mandatory hospital and department specific orientation requirements, attendance at necessary training sessions, a yearly review of each acupuncturist's clinical experience, competencies, and/or quality assurance data. A written review will be sent to the Zakim Center office to be included in the acupuncturist's file.

PROVISION OF ACUPUNCTURE SERVICES

A. Physician/Dentist Referral

    An acupuncturist may commence acupuncture treatments upon a patient only after a referral or a written diagnosis has been completed by a physician or dentist who is a member of the DFCI medical staff.

B. Location of Acupuncture Services

    Acupuncture treatments will be provided to ambulatory patients on the eleventh floor of the Dana Building and when necessary in other outpatient or inpatient settings.

C. Acupuncture Treatments Acupuncture treatments shall be performed in compliance with the Massachusetts Regulations Governing the Practice of Acupuncture (243 CMR 5.00).

D. Temporary Privileges

Table 7.2 (continued)

<u>Non-MDs</u>

For compassionate reasons, temporary privileges may be granted to a patient's own Acupuncturist who does not have DFCI privileges. The following documents will need to be on file:

1. Copy of the practitioner's Massachusetts license;
2. Proof of malpractice insurance coverage;
3. Letter of reference from a peer;
4. Signed approval sheet by the Medical Director of the Leonard P. Zakim Center for Integrated Therapies or his designee.

Temporary privileges will be granted for one case only and will be terminated upon the completion of the patient's treatment.

<u>MDs</u>

Medical doctors must request temporary privileges as outlined in the DFCI bylaws.
APPROVED: MSEC:

---

to perform it based on their scope of practice. As a result, the Reiki clinical policy states that one must be a MA-licensed RN in order to perform Reiki at DFCI. Unlike acupuncture providers, massage therapists are not licensed by Massachusetts, so even more discourse was required to find a starting point for competency assessment and to create policies that assured highly qualified staff (see Table 7.3). Table 7.4

Table 7.3 Dana-Farber Cancer Institute Massage Therapy Policy

PURPOSE: To provide Massage Therapy for pediatric and adult patients in the clinical areas.

SCOPE: This policy applies to all DFCI staff who are trained and involved with patient care.
OBJECTIVES:

1. To promote relaxation and sense of comfort
2. To improve circulation
3. To alter the perception of pain, therefore alleviating discomfort
4. To decrease anxiety and depression, and increase alertness

POLICY: To provide a safe massage for adult and pediatric patients.
    Massage can be performed by any registered nurse.
    Therapeutic massage requires further training and can be done by a massage therapist who has completed an approved program of atleast 500 hours of training and who are licensed to practice massage in the City of Boston.

PROCEDURE: Massage Therapy involves touch and different techniques to manipulate the soft tissue of the body. Massage can involve only part of the body full body massage. It can be done through one's clothing or on the exposed skin. It can be done on a special massage chair, in a bed or on a massage table. Massage is supported by research and is practiced as an adjunct to conventional care.

    Before giving a massage it is important to review the patients medical history. Contraindications for massage are that massage should not be done over any area of inflammation, infection, altered skin integrity, rashes, areas of bruising, trauma or surgery. Massage should not be done at a tumor site, areas of edema, if blood counts are low, thrombosis, or abnormal sensations. Massage should not be done over or near any in dwelling catheters.

(continued)

Table 7.3 (continued)

Massage is always individualized and a session may last 30-60 minutes. In general neonates, children, the elderly, those with psychiatric disorders, and those who are debilitated will require a lighter touch and briefer session.

Procedures:

1. Review patient medical history and current health status.
2. Explain the procedure.
3. Patient is placed in supportive position.
4. Patient's body temperature should be maintained during the massage. Areas not being massaged should be covered for warmth and privacy.
5. Touch should be light, smooth, rhythmical and relaxed.
6. If patient has lymphedema contact primary oncologist about referal to therapist for specific treatment.
7. If patient is undergoing radiation therapy, massage at the radiation site is contraindicated.
8. Adjustment may be made to the amount of pressure and occasionally delay in massage for patients at risk for low blood counts.
9. Communicate with the patient during the session about comfort.
10. Document the procedure and patient feedback. Massage can effect a change in patient condition that needs to be recorded.
11. Hands should be disinfected with a waterless hand agent before and after patient contact. Soap and water should be used only when hands are visibly soiled.
12. A water-filled lotion warmer maybe used. The warmer should be emptied and cleaned with alcohol or asepti-wipes after use at mid-day and at the end of the day. The entire massage lotion bottle should be wiped off with alcohol or an Asepti wipe after each use.
13. The massage therapist is supervised by the Medical Director or his/her designee of the Zakim Center.

References:

1. Board of Registration in Nursing, Commonwealth of Mass. (1997) *Advisory ruling: Holistic Nursing Practice and Complementary Therapies.* Mass. General Laws (GL), Chapter 30A, Section 8, and Chapter 112, Section 80B
2. Fritz, S. (1995). *Mosby's Fundamental of Therapeutic Massage.* St. Louis: Mosby Lifeline.
3. MacDonald, Gayle, (1999)*Medicine Hands, Massage Therapy for People with Cancer,* Findhorn Press.
4. Tappan, F. (1988). *Healing Massage Techniques: Holistic, Classic And Emerging Methods,* Norwalk, CT, Appleton and Lange.

Approved: Zakim Executive Committee
Date: April 2002

Rev.: Zakim Executive Committee
Date: March 2005

---

represents the competency evaluation currently performed annually by all massage therapists at DFCI.

In establishing clinic operations, there was also much to consider.

- Would a referral be needed?
- Where would practitioners document their notes?

- Would patients pay for services or would insurance companies be billed?
- How much treatment space would be needed?
- Who would book appointments?
- How would the DFCI community be informed about the CAM clinical services?

A treatment room in the Hematology Malignancy Clinic was secured that could be used part-time a few days per week. Although the space was small and had limited availability, it was centrally located in the middle of a very busy clinic. Offering acupuncture and Reiki in this clinic was true integration. Clinicians and patients were able to interact with the complementary therapy providers, and patients were able to get CAM services alongside their conventional treatment.

7.4 Documentation and Scheduling of Integrative Therapies

Today, providers document procedures in the same medical record as the rest of the clinical team. Practitioners are required to use templates in a modified SOAP format. Acupuncturists and other CAM therapists write in English and use words and abbreviations that the conventional medical providers understand and have been approved by Dana-Farber. Notes are written directly into the EMR, and Zakim Center providers have full access to the entire record, greatly increasing communication between providers. Patients can schedule appointments with any of the CAM practice coordinators at DFCI and do not need to come to the Zakim Center to do so. Schedules are built into the same scheduling system as all other Institute services.

Physician-initiated referrals are not required for any CAM services, with the exception of Integrative Medicine/Oncology Consultations. Most requests come from patient self-referrals, family, and clinical staff other than physicians. After a patient schedules his or her appointment, the primary oncologist is contacted by email and asked if the patient is medically eligible for the service based on defined medical and psychosocial. An example of such an email is seen in Fig. 7.1. DFCI clinicians respond about their patient's eligibility by email, and 95% of the time they do so within 24 h. This greatly enhances the communication between Zakim Center providers and DFCI clinicians and often opens a dialog for the Zakim provider to hear firsthand from the oncologist about the patient's condition and assures all involved that the services implemented are supervised and safe.

Intake forms and evaluations are now completed after all services: group and individual, educational, clinical, and research. Reports go back to the oncologist or care team if there is a significant finding or significant report of a new symptom. Our program is monitored for quality assurance via several quality indicators including adverse events, clinic volume, financial assistance requests, capacity, and the means by which patients hear about our offerings. Patient and staff satisfaction evaluations are also performed periodically, and techniques to effectively measure the benefits and risks of new and existing programs are continuously introduced and evaluated.

Table 7.4 Competency Evaluation form

Dana-Farber Cancer Institute
Massage Therapist Competencies
Name: _____ **Date of Hire:** _____

Methods of Validation Return completed form to:
OBS – observation
RTD – return demonstration
DSC - Discussion

Skill	Validation Method	Date Completed	Orientee Initials	Preceptor Initials
Basic Patient Care				
Wears appropriate attire or lab coat during practice.				
Introduces self to patient and escorts them to the room.				
Checks ID band before treatment.				
Talks to patient about medical history, pertinent information and appropriate massage procedures, modifications and expectations.				
Acknowledges patient requests, questions or needs before and after the massage.				
Assists patients in positioning or getting on/off table if needed.				
Keeps patient comfortable, (i.e. checks room temperature, need for pillow support) and maintains proper draping at all times.				
Maintains good hygiene and infection control at all times:				
• Maintains proper hand-washing techniques before and after each massage.				
• Changes linens, pillowcases, towels used for every patient.				
• Washes or uses approved disinfectant for bottles and lotion tips after every use.				
• Wipes counter tops, face cradles, doorknobs at anytime oil/lotion contamination occurs and at the end of the day.				
• Gathers linens and puts in soiled linen bag after each patient and prepares it for collection at the end of the day.				
Maintains patient privacy and confidentiality at all times.				
Information Gathering/Documentation				
Reviews eligibility letter for 1st time patients.				
Reviews records for medical, physical and psychosocial history and notes of other caregivers.				
Contacts other caregivers as necessary if there are any questions or concerns about the patient.				

Reviews laboratory results at each visit.
Develops plan of care with patient for each visit and for long-term goals.
Documents date/time of massage, pertinent information and patient response in the medical records.

Scope of Practice
Demonstrates the ability to discuss the scientific basis for massage therapy.
Describes the uses of massage for the cancer patient.
Describes contraindications for massage in cancer patients (i.e. risk factors due to effects of the cancer, effects of treatment, organ involvement).
Demonstrates commonly used techniques (effleurage, petrissage, vibration, percussion, passive body).
Demonstrates the ability to modify the massage techniques and components (i.e. speed, pressure, duration) on a case to case basis.
Demonstrates the ability to suggest self-care techniques or other integrative modalities that can be helpful to patient.
Understands various measurements of psychological and physiological outcomes.
Keeps updated with latest research or workshops in the use of massage especially in the cancer setting.

Information Systems
Demonstrates working knowledge of Outlook Email.Created by Information Systems.
Demonstrates working knowledge of IDX, as appropriate.
Demonstrates working knowledge of LMR as appropriate.
Comments:

Signatures   Date
Orientee: _____
Preceptor: _____
Manager: _____
Medical Director: _____

7.5 Zakim Center Collaborations

From the very beginning of this grass-roots effort, involving the local healthcare community was crucial. Most of the Boston-area experts in complementary therapies were not based at DFCI, and many of them were eager to offer their expertise and assistance in program development. Collaborating with local academic institutions and community organizations has continued to serve the Center well. Through

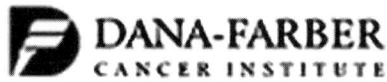

Leonard P. Zakim Center for Integrated Therapies

Acupuncture Eligibility Letter Template

Hello **Dr. SMITH**,

One of your patients, **JOHN DOE, MRN: 123456**, has requested an acupuncture visit. I tentatively scheduled him/her for **Wednesday, April 3rd**, pending your approval. The following is a guideline used to determine patient eligibility for acupuncture:
At this time, acupuncture treatment is NOT recommended to cancer patients with the following conditions:

a. Absolute neutrophil count (ANC) less than 500/ml
b. Platelet count less than 25,000/ml
c. Altered mental state
d. Clinically significant cardiac arrhythmias
e. Other unstable medical conditions (case-by-case consideration)

The following conditions may benefit from acupuncture treatment:

a. Chronic pain (e.g.cancer-related, post operative, musculo-skeletal)
b. Headaches(e.g. tension headaches or migraine headaches)
c. Depression and anxiety
d. Chemotherapy-induced nausea and vomiting
e. Low WBC count
f. Immune deficiency
g. Constipation
h. Insomnia
i. Various musculo-skeletal pain

I'd appreciate you letting me know if your patient, **JOHN DOE, MRN:**, is eligible for acupuncture by replying to this email. In case you'd like more information on acupuncture, I'm attaching a link to the NIH Consensus Statement on Acupuncture. http://odp.od.nih.gov/consensus/cons/107/107_statement.htm

Thank you,

The information transmitted in this E-mail is intended only for the person or entity to which it is addressed and may contain confidential and/or privileged material. Any review, retransmission, dissemination or other use of or taking of any action in reliance upon, this information by persons or entities other than the intended recipient is prohibited. If you received this E-mail in error, please contact the sender and delete the material from any computer.

Approved: Zakim Center Executive Committee
Date: December, 2000
Revised: March, 2005

Fig. 7.1 Acupuncture Eligibility Letter

a research study with community providers, Qigong was offered to eligible patients with breast cancer, prostate cancer, and/or chronic lymphocytic leukemia. Community involvement also helped in identifying and developing a number of other therapies group programs, including music therapy, journaling, and expressive arts therapy.

Private foundation funding was also of great benefit. It allowed us to offer writing workshops, a mediation program, and a dance program. Productive mutual arrangements were established with Lesley University, Massachusetts College of Pharmacy and Allied Health (MCP), and the world-renowned Berklee College of Music. Through our arrangements with Lesley, for instance, an expressive arts therapy program was developed with funding by a private foundation. The Zakim Center provided the oncology expertise, Lesley the therapy skills, and patients experienced a direct benefit from the collaboration.

As word of its services spread, the Zakim Center continued to grow. Information sheets for patients on herbs and supplementation were written in collaboration with The MCP, and today nutritional services are a large component of the center. In 2001, a pharmacy student shadow program was initiated, and three or four fifth-year doctoral students now spend time in the Zakim Center each semester observing complementary therapies. Their curriculum includes assessing the actions of acupuncture for post-chemotherapy nausea and the decrease of anti-nausea medication. The pharmacy students bring their knowledge to our Zakim Center clinicians by offering information about the medications patients are taking and herb–drug interactions, making this a mutually beneficial arrangement.

In 1999, a Health Psychology student intern from MCP began in the Zakim Center for 10 h per week on various projects, including coordinating complementary therapy fairs, organizing mind-body workshops, and developing patient resources. While at the Zakim Center, the intern attends center meetings and interacts with the integrative medicine providers and patients. In addition to these programs, and in hope of securing more, an information packet on the Zakim Center was produced describing the work of the center and providing information on CAM.

The collaboration with the Berklee College of Music began in 2000. The Music Therapy Department at Berklee needed clinical sites for student training, while the Zakim Center desired to offer music therapy to DFCI patients, family members, and staff without raising additional funds. Led by the Chair of the Music Therapy Department at Berklee, a music therapy program began at DFCI in which drop-in music therapy sessions were offered in conference rooms. They continue to this day, and some have lent themselves to research projects.

7.6 Growth of the Zakim Center

When the center officially opened in November 2000, mind-body therapies, Reiki, nutrition, and acupuncture were delivered in a borrowed exam room in the Adult Hematology Malignancies clinic. A lengthy waiting list soon began, and it was evident after only 6 months that the patients' needs were not being met. Once the limited individual clinical services were initiated, patients and staff wanted more, more than funding or space permitted. But in order to add services, several questions had to be addressed:

- Are DFCI patients interested in this service?
- Is the DFCI administration interested in it?
- Is it safe?
- Is it effective?
- Does it fit into the Institute's mission?
- How can the program be offered at minimal cost?
- Who will coordinate it?
- Is there an on-site location available for this service?

Numerous phone calls and emails were received from CAM practitioners in the Greater Boston community and beyond who wanted to help and work at DFCI. In order to effectively consider and respond to these inquiries and offers, however, concrete information from each community provider who wanted to offer their services at DFCI was needed. A brief proposal format was created which included individual resumes, description of topic/therapy, target audience, rationale, budget, and resource needs. Additional staff could not be hired without additional funding, so alternative mechanisms had to be explored.

A staff survey helped the Zakim Center find out who at DFCI had been trained as a complementary therapy provider. Those who were already trained to do one of the needed therapies were contacted and asked if they could work it into their regular workdays to offer these programs or services to patients. Responses were strong and positive, and as a result, several programs such as Yoga for staff and patients and mind-body therapy workshops for patients were implemented at no charge to participants and at minimal cost to the Zakim Center.

Clinical operations in CAM began in the Jimmy Fund Clinic (JFC), Dana-Farber's pediatric program, in 2001. An integrative medicine physician was hired to work with the JFC Medical Director to offer integrative medicine consultations and to work closely with a pediatrician and the Center for Holistic Pediatric Education and Research (CHPER) at Children's Hospital, Boston, another Harvard facility just down the street where DFCI inpatients stay.

On top of this, additional adult clinical space at Dana-Farber became available in December 2001, and a clinical suite of three treatment rooms and a practitioner office were constructed on one of the Institute's clinical service floors.

The Zakim Center continued to expand with more clinical, educational, and research offerings. Our first acupuncture research study, a National Center for Complementary and Alternative Medicine (NCCAM)-funded R21 pilot study, began enrolling patients in 2002, the same year a clinical research coordinator was hired. A physician was brought on board from the NCI via an interagency personnel agreement, allowing the center to expand its professional education program and offer integrative medicine consultation to medical staff. Integrative medical consultations offer comprehensive medical history assessment and answer specific questions about herb/drug interactions, treatment side effects, and so on, and adding them had a tremendous impact on the center's clinic volume. In just one year, the Zakim Center patient encounters doubled from 778 in 2001 to more than 1600 in 2002.

With its core patient numbers strong, the Zakim Center focus between 2003 and 2005 was on expanding availability for individual services, offering additional group programs, and bringing services to patients who could not come to the ambulatory clinic. Credentialing providers to offer in-patient services began, and soon thereafter, services began on in-patient units at partnering Brigham and Women's Hospital.

Today, there are four acupuncturists and four massage therapists offering clinical services to DFCI's patients. Integrative Medicine/Oncology consultations, integrative nutrition counseling, therapeutic touch, Reiki, and mind-body therapies are available for adult and pediatric patients. Music therapy group and individual sessions are available to pediatric patients in a dedicated treatment room in the JFC. Qigong classes are offered weekly and Yoga, expressive arts therapy, and meditation programs continue to be part of the center's group program schedule. Reiki and massage therapy are offered on the in-patient units at Brigham and Women's, and a music therapy service is also being developed for in-patients. Total clinic volume for the Zakim Center has grown to over 5000 encounters per year, and cancer patients from all DFCI partner hospitals including Massachusetts General Hospital and the Faulkner Hospital are eligible to come to the Institute to partake in center services. Two other partner hospitals are planning a "Zakim Center" in their facilities, so that their patients can benefit from on-site medically supervised integrative therapies.

7.7 Financials

Affordability and accessibility have been key issues from the outset at the Zakim Center.

In developing their action plan for the center, leadership expected that financial support would not come from hospital operating funds. "Team Lenny" participants took part in two of DFCI fundraising events, the Boston Marathon JFW and the Pan Massachusetts Challenge (PMC), a 192-mile bike ride. Together these teams have brought in hundreds of thousands of dollars to support Zakim Center services and programs; currently, philanthropic donations fund 70% of center services. Individual gifts and other Zakim Center-directed special events bring in the major income of the center. Philanthropy cannot cover all expenses, however, so a reduced fee is charged for each of the services. A fee can be billed to insurance for some services such as integrative medicine and integrative nutritional consultations, but few insurance companies will reimburse hospitals for other CAM services such as acupuncture, massage, Reiki, therapeutic touch, and individual music therapy. DFCI has always set fees at a reduced market rate, so the therapies are more affordable for patients. As an additional measure, a special encounter form/receipt was developed that contains all the current ICD and CPT codes, location, DFCI Tax ID, provider signature line, and other necessary information a patient needs to submit his or her receipt to an insurance company for potential reimbursement.

In order to make our program affordable and accessible to all, a financial assistance mechanism was put in place for those who cannot afford the fee. Any patient is eligible to apply for a discount via an application that DFCI financial counselors review. Because the fee will still be too costly for some patients, those who are on Medicaid or "Free Care" can partake in six free treatments per therapy per calendar year.

There is no fee for any group program, and most of these, including mind-body therapies, expressive arts therapy, meditation, Yoga, Qigong, and music therapy, are available to families and staff as well as patients.

Because DFCI does not collect money at the time of service including co-payments, except for pharmacy needs, a system had to be created in which a patient can pay for a Zakim Center visit and then return to clinic for treatment. Figure 7.2 demonstrates the patient flow through DFCI for integrative therapies.

In establishing systems and operations, communication was crucial between the Zakim Center, and Dana-Farber Patient Accounts, staff, Financial Counselors, Operations and Nurse Managers, and Resource Centers. Differences in operations from other services offered by the Institute created a need for us to constantly evaluate and re-evaluate our operations and program offerings, so that patient and provider needs continue to be met in the most efficient and effective manner possible.

In 2003, a group of Harvard Business School students evaluated the Zakim Center program. They worked free of charge as part of their curriculum and performed an extensive analysis that includes several recommendations that were later implemented. These included ways to better market our services, another good example of community resources helping benefit the center.

An Operations Workgroup for integrative therapies was formed at Dana-Farber late in 2003 to focus on streamlining operations. This group was comprised of the center's Program Manager, the Director of Business Administration for Nursing and Patient Care Service, the Director of Access Management, the Director of Patient Accounting, and adult and pediatric nurse managers. Meeting regularly and the group sought to develop the best operational systems possible.

As previously stated, communication, outreach and marketing, and community relations are very important for the integration of CAM into Dana-Farber's lifestyle. There are regular meetings with the multidisciplinary care disease centers to determine what their needs are and discuss how the Zakim Center can best fit into their mission. Monthly clinical practice meetings are held in which patient issues are discussed with the center's medical director and clinical team. Practitioners present case studies on compelling patients that they feel would be an important learning experience for the team. The patient's entire medical care team is invited to this meeting so that a true integrative medicine case discussion ensues.

7 Integrative Oncology

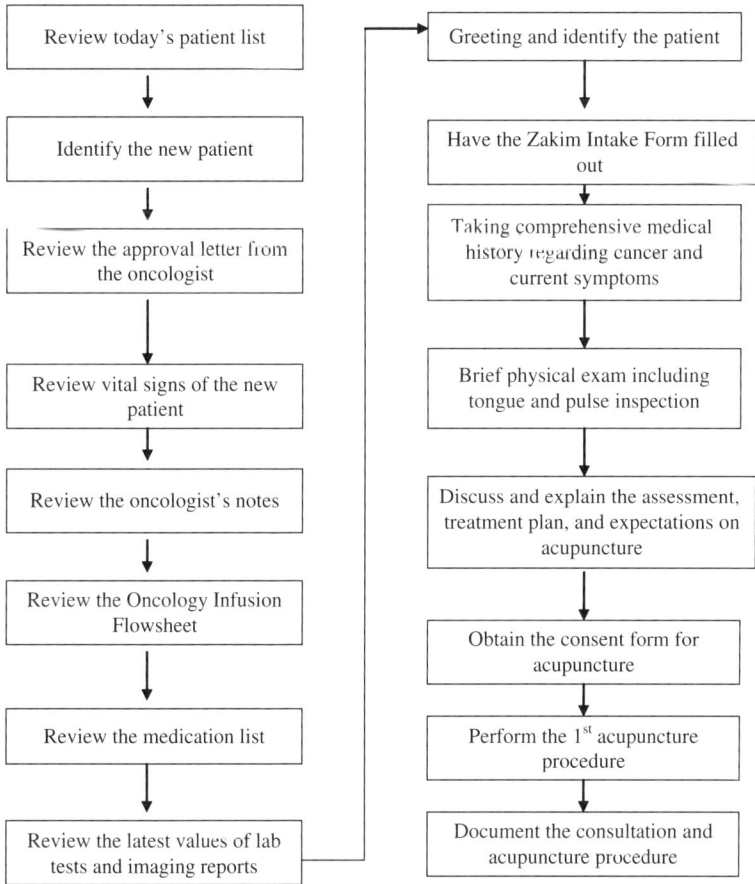

Fig. 7.2 Initial acupuncture consultation and treatment flow chart at Zakim Center, Dana-Farber Cancer Institute.

7.8 Creating an Integrative Education Program for Patients and Families, Physicians, Nurses, and Researchers

Patients and their advocates are aware that many cancer diagnoses are chronic and incurable. Often seeking out CAM information can result in coming to terms with illness and controlling symptoms. Medical and scientific research promotes discussion of CAM practice in a non-judgmental, legally responsible, and ethical manner. This leads to patients making decisions on how to improve their healthcare.

As an outgrowth of the strategic planning initiatives of the original Complementary Therapy Task Force, a subcommittee devoted to education was formed.

Meeting monthly, it was chaired by the director of Patient Family Education who also served as Chair of the CAM Division of the NCI Cancer Patient Education Network (CPEN). The mission of the interdisciplinary subcommittee members was twofold: to provide and foster open communication between local providers and patients, and to develop a series of lectures and written teaching sheets for the Dana-Farber community. Collaborating with NCI/CPEN and the Longwood Herbal Task Force, the education subcommittee conducted a comprehensive review of the literature for evidence-based research: specifically, safe, noninvasive complementary therapy practices with few potential negative side effects.

In March 1998, at the task force's introductory lecture for patients, families and professional staff, given by Dr. David Eisenberg, a teaching sheet on complementary therapies was distributed. Shortly thereafter, the Integrative Medical Alliance (IMA) was formed, a fast growing community of CAM practitioners in the Boston area, which is now an active independent non-profit corporation. One of the IMA's functions was to create a list of potential speakers and plan programs for staff and patients. A series of monthly lectures followed and a teaching sheet was written in plain language for each session to define the modality and serve as a starting point for open discussion on proven research and known side effects (Table 7.5). An evaluation form was developed and distributed at each lecture (Table 7.6).

Table 7.5 Dana-Farber Cancer Institute Lectures and Teaching Sheets Written Under the Complementary and Alternative Medicine Domains of National Center for Complementary and Alternative Medicine

Alternative medical systems: Ayurveda Medicine, Homeopathy, Traditional Chinese Medicine/Acupuncture
Mind-body interventions: Aromatherapy, Focusing, Guided Imagery, Meditation, Music and Sound Therapy, Pilates, Relaxation Response, Walking the Labyrinth, Yoga
Manipulative and body-based methods: Chiropractic, Physical Exercise, Shiatsu Massage/Acupressure, Therapeutic Massage
Biologically based therapies: Antioxidants, Co-Enzyme Q10, Vitamins/Minerals, Food Substance (Mushroom), Coriolus Versicolor (PSK), Herbs, Milk Thistle
Energy Therapies: Reflexology, Reiki, Qigong, Therapeutic Touch, Zero Balancing

Table 7.6

A summary of attendance of lectures given to patients, families and staff:		
	No.	Topic
Least attended	6	Massage
Most attended	79	Healthy eating while living with cancer
Mean audience size	39	
Most staff attended	55	Nutrients and oncogenesis
Most patient/families	59	Feng Shui
Most frequently requested lecture		Yoga class
How do patients hear about programs?	52%	Flyers/Publications
	20%	Staff
	5%	M.D.
Most frequent recommendation on evaluation		More case studies
		More time for Q & A

The Zakim Center education subcommittee added this disclaimer on each teaching sheet:

> By making this information available, neither the Patient Family Education Council nor Dana-Farber Cancer Institute makes any recommendations or promises, or guarantees the effectiveness of this complementary therapy. For any serious condition please contact your doctor before trying any new therapy. If you do decide to try this modality of therapy, please inform your doctor or nurse so all practitioners can work together to help you in the healing process.

Sufficient patient-family feedback and comments continue to be positive. A monthly class on introduction to complementary therapies for adults was implemented, and later, a similar class for parents of pediatric patients began. An additional educational opportunity occurs at the annual DFCI CAM Fair open to the public, patients, families, and staff. Opportunities for learning, demonstrations, and actual interactions with practitioners have all been met with high satisfaction.

7.8.1 Professional Education

Professional education is an integral part of incorporating complementary offerings into conventional patient care at DFCI. Many practicing oncologists, nurses, social workers, and other health professionals working on a multi-disciplinary healthcare team have had little or no prior curriculum or training regarding CAM therapies such as massage, acupuncture, and herbs or dietary supplements. As a result, they feel that they lack sufficient familiarity to advise their patients.

Despite the high CAM usage by cancer patients [2–5], there is often no discussion or mutual understanding between patients and their physicians about these offerings. Sometimes, patients are unaware of certain therapies that could benefit them, whereas in other cases, patients use unsupervised therapies with potentially serious implications. It is well-documented in the medical literature that communication between patients and their physicians regarding CAM use often does not occur; this finding is not specific to cancer patients [6]. Even more alarmingly, oncologists and cancer patients are shown to have discrepant views on CAM that contribute to this communication gap [7].

It is important to have acceptance of integrative medicine by a hospital's medical staff in order to better serve its cancer patients. On a national level, having sources of federally funded, peer-reviewed CAM research by the National Institutes of Health has expanded medical professionals' education and knowledge about these modalities. Furthermore, research has helped to establish the legitimacy of CAM as the subject of scientific inquiry, advancing the field via greater cooperation between clinical investigators and CAM practitioners.

The field of CAM and integrative oncology itself is evolving, as more evidence-based information becomes available regarding the safety, efficacy, and risks and benefits of already-studied therapies. For all these reasons, it is important to have both introductory and ongoing educational opportunities for the entire clinical staff, as well as educational resources available for staff use.

In response to the need for CAM professional education at DFCI, members of the Zakim Center staff have incorporated several ongoing programs and activities. For the past 3 years, an introductory academic CAM lecture has been provided to new fellows as part of their core academic curriculum. Additionally, the Zakim Center provides periodic presentations at staff meetings of Dana-Farber's various Multidisciplinary Care Centers (MCC), for example, which specialize in breast cancer, head and neck cancer, neuro-oncology, and so on. These short presentations have incorporated a combination of core information on the Zakim Center and IM as well as recently published medical literature and/or case studies tailored to issues faced by that care center's particular patient population. Making these presentations more appealing is that a number of them are approved for Continuing Medical Education (CME) and Continuing Education Units (CEUs). All new staff are introduced to the Zakim Center in the New Staff Orientation.

A number of additional measures also help to educate the DFCI community about IM. The Institute provides a number of reliable databases that can be accessed by physicians and other staff regarding information about the benefits and side effects of herbs and botanicals. Dana-Farber has a site license for the Natural Medicines Comprehensive Database, a subscription resource with evidence-based information on herbs and supplements that can be accessed at any DFCI computer. Additionally, the IM consultation service provides educational information and guidance to a patient's oncology team through discussions and clinical notes.

Similarly, as part of fulfilling its mission to cancer patients, the Zakim Center staff is dedicated to providing ongoing professional education so that clinicians can advise patients knowledgeably on a truly integrative approach to their care, combining the best practices of conventional treatment along with complementary therapies.

7.9 Development of a Research Program

DFCI is a world-renowned cancer patient care research institute, so the Zakim Center staff knew from the beginning that conducting research would be an important step in becoming part of the Institute culture. It was decided to focus research on the clinical services offered at the center, such as acupuncture, Reiki, and group therapy programs such as music and Qigong. We tapped the expertise of the master clinicians and practitioners who offered the clinical services; the first pilot study performed, for instance, was on a patient's immunological activity, quality of life, and physical status in connection with a modified exercise program and Qigong in patients with breast cancer, prostate cancer, and/or chronic lymphocytic leukemia [8]. The study was a combined effort of the Department of Hematological Oncology, the Zakim Center, the Department of Rehabilitation at Brigham & Women's Hospital, and Social Medicine at Harvard Medical School and began on the assumption that moderate physical exercise and stress reduction may have a beneficial effect on immunity, Qigong is a Chinese practice that incorporates meditation and exercise, and preliminary studies suggested that an increase in the proportion of CD4-positive helper lymphocytes was present in healthy volunteers practicing Qigong. With the support of a Dana Foundation grant, patients were randomly assigned to Qigong or modified exercise as their initial experience on a weekly basis. Both programs involved 90 min of structured activity. Blood samples were obtained at base line and approximately 90–120 min after completion of the program. Outcome measurements included the psychosocial instruments (POMS, FACT-SP, and brief COPE). Goniometry measurements were obtained prior to the first session and following the second session. Participants included asymptomatic patients who were not currently doing structured intensive exercise. The study employed a crossover design with each patient acting as his or her own control.

In this first study, our clinicians realized the difficulty in performing complementary therapy research. Of 121 patients eligible for this intervention, 23% had conflicts that precluded participation. Six percent were interested but had already exercised too much, while 59% were non-responsive to the request and ultimately just 12% (15 patients) agreed to participate. Patient recruitment and study completion were challenging aspects of this trial, but in the end, it did prove feasible.

The next project, an R-21 funded by the NCCAM at the NIH (NCCAM/NIH) [9], took advantage of the expertise of our traditional Chinese medicine-trained acupuncturists. The goal was to determine the feasibility of studying acupuncture in an ambulatory population of seriously ill advanced cancer patients and to assess the utility of various quality-of-life instruments. This pilot study met its goal of enrolling 40 patients with advanced ovarian or breast cancer. Each patient received 12 sessions of acupuncture, twice a week for the first 4 weeks, then once a week for the next 4 weeks. A standardized protocol of pre-selected points was used, with designated symptom-specific points also used as needed. The quality-of-life questionnaires were completed at five time points—pre treatment, week 4, week 8 (the end of treatment), week 9, and week 12. The regimen was considered feasible if 50% of the patients completed the 8-week treatment. This study demonstrated feasibility and there were no adverse events from the protocol. This pilot also showed some clinical benefit, with patients reporting positive benefits, both by report of reduced symptoms and improvement in quality of life at one or more sessions. After the study's completion, some patients chose to continue acupuncture treatments as part of their clinical care.

In researching Chinese literature, the traditional Chinese medicine acupuncturists also found 11 clinical studies that suggested a beneficial effect of acupuncture for chemotherapy-induced leukopenia. This led to the development of a randomized clinical trial funded by the NCCAM/NIH to determine whether acupuncture could indeed reduce the neutropenic effect of chemotherapy [10]. In preparing for this research study, the acupuncturists had to develop a "sham acupuncture" procedure. This was a learning experience for the practitioners, none of whom had done sham acupuncture before.

The first three clinical research studies brought together the Zakim Center's practitioners with "traditional" clinical staff and involved several of the MCCs at DFCI. Additional investigations include studies on the effect of Qigong on the mood and cortisol levels in breast cancer, the use of music therapy with metastatic breast cancer, and a feasibility study assessing the effect of two complementary therapies, either relaxation response with cognitive restructuring or Reiki versus a control group, in men receiving radiation therapy for prostate cancer. The enrollment phase for this three-arm, randomized study has been active and is expected to reach its goal of 60 patients.

To this point, the center has avoided carrying out clinical studies on herbs and botanicals, because of the lack of standardization of the products and the difficulty that colleagues have had previously in studying herbs such as PC-SPES in prostate cancer [11].

In advancing the strategy of further research in integrative therapies, the research leadership at DFCI decided to review the entire Institute's research with integrative therapies. To gather such a portfolio, a memorandum was sent to all Dana-Farber scientists and clinicians requesting information on any research they had conducted on herbs, botanicals, antioxidants, nutritional supplements, exercise, mind-body, acupuncture, and other complementary therapies. These studies include pre-clinical, clinical or basic science research, as well as studies of mechanism of action. A portfolio of CAM research at DFCI resulted helping to develop a comprehensive research plan on integrative therapies throughout the Institute.

7.10 Concluding Thoughts

In the face of one's mortality, people confront incredible choices. The awareness of a cancer diagnosis forces every person to review their life and priorities. In November 2005, the Leonard P. Zakim Center for Integrative Therapies celebrated its fifth anniversary with a complementary therapy fair and a keynote lecture by Dr. Ralph Snyderman, Emeritus Chancellor of Duke University, and Professor of Medicine at Duke University School of Medicine. The joyous, well-attended event would have greatly pleased the first major advocate for IM at DFCI. Lenny Zakim lived his life to serve others and to find ways to bridge the divide between many different groups of people, recognizing the importance of working collectively toward shared goals. Through years of rigorous experimental cancer treatment, months of decreased energy and enjoyment, weeks, days, and minutes of pain and disability, Lenny continued to follow this path and credo. His journey with cancer inspired him to make the road less painful for those who would follow after, and he planted the seeds that made the Leonard P. Zakim Center for Integrative Therapies a reality at DFCI. Now it is hoped that through our experiences, we can help other cancer centers achieve a similar vision.

References

1. Complementary Therapies: Empowering the Cancer Patient, Dana-Farber Cancer Institute, ISBN No. 1-890921-B, Xenejenex Health Care Communication.
2. Cassileth B, Deng G. Complementary and alternative therapies for cancer. Oncologist 2004, 9, 80–89.
3. Richardson M, Sanders T, Palmer J, et al. Complementary/alternative medicine use in a comprehensive cancer center and the implications on oncology. J Clin Oncol 2000, 18, 2505–2514.
4. DiGianni L, Garber J. Winer, E. Complementary and alternative medicine use among women with breast cancer. J Clin Oncol 2002, 20, 34s–38s.
5. Boon H, Westlakek S, Gray R, Fleshner N, Gavin A, Brown J, Goel V. Use of complementary/alternative medicine by men diagnosed with prostate cancer: prevalence and characteristics. Urology 2003, 62, 849–853.
6. Eisenberg D. Perceptions about complementary therapies relative to conventional therapies among adults who use both: results from a national survey. Ann Intern Med 2001, 135, 344–351.
7. Richardson MA, Mâsse LC, Nanny K, Sanders C. Discrepant views of oncologists and cancer patients on complementary/alternative medicine. Support Cancer Care 2004, 12, 797–804.
8. Doherty-Gilman A, Richardson P, Neuberg D, Momtaz P, Bears J, Odaka B, Rones R, Kerr C, Nazir F, Ott MJ, Rosenthal DS, Freedman A. A Pilot Study of Immunologic Activity, Quality of Life, and Physical Status in Connection with Two Exercise Programs (Modified Exercise and Qigong) in Patients with Breast Cancer, Prostate Cancer, or Chronic Lymphocytic Leukemia (CLL). Plenary Synopsis from Society for Integrative Oncology (SIO) meeting, Journal of Society of Integrative Oncology, December 2005, 3 (4), 133–135.
9. Dean-Clower E, Doherty-Gilman A, Baker F, Kaw C, Donoria W, Manola J, DellaCroce A, Sugumar A, Ohiri K, Geng A, Rosenthal DS. Effect of Acupuncture on the Pain, Nausea, and Quality of Life of Patient with Advanced Cancer. Plenary Synopsis from Society for Integrative Oncology (SIO) meeting, Journal of Society of Integrative Oncology, December 2005, 3 (4), 130–131.
10. Lu W, Hu D, Dean-Clower E, Matulonis U, Rosenthal DS. A Systematic Review on Acupuncture Trials for Chemotherapy-Induced Leukopenia, Plenary Synopsis from SIO meeting. Plenary Synopsis from Society for Integrative Oncology (SIO) meeting, Journal of Society of Integrative Oncology, December 2005, 3 (4), 135–137.
11. Oh WK, Kantoff PW, Weinberg V, Jones G, Rini BI, Derynck MK, Bok R, Smith MR, Bubley GJ, Rosen RT, DiPaola RS, Small EJ. Prospective, multicenter, randomized phase II trial of the herbal supplement, PC-SPES, and diethylstilbestrol in patients with androgen-independent prostate cancer. J Clin Oncol 2004, Sep 15, 22 (18), 3705–3712.

Chapter 8
The Johns Hopkins Complementary and Integrative Medicine Service

Kathleen Menten, Sanghoon Lee, and Adrian S. Dobs

Contents

8.1	Introduction	106
8.2	Clinical Service Initial Stage Development Process	106
8.3	Practical Aspects in Planning a Complementary and Integrative Medicine Service	108
8.4	Services Now Being Provided	110
8.5	Administration of the CIM Service	113
8.6	Financial Aspects	115
8.7	Education Programs	117
8.8	Case Study	118
8.9	Challenges Faced by the Complementary and Integrative Medicine Service	119
8.10	Conclusions/Summary	120
References		121

Abstract The Johns Hopkins Complementary and Integrative Medical Service was developed to provide patients with opportunities to broaden their conventional care. Beginning with a research focus, further funding was obtained to begin a clinical service. This provides the patients with procedures that address quality of life issues while they are receiving conventional treatments. Providing these services under the auspices of the hospital helps patients feel more comfortable. In this chapter we describe the essential steps needed for the planning, development and implementation of a program. Our service needed to comply with the existing organizational parameters of the institution. Initial stages require a multidisciplinary planning process that addresses the following issues: patient population, employed practitioners vs. independent contractors, risk/benefit ratio for services, standards of care, policies and procedures, referral requirements, and documentation requirements, credentialing, billing and form development. We have had multiple challenges including acceptance by the medical community and financial pressures. Although the road

---

A. Dobs
Professor of Medicine and Oncology, Division of Endocrinology and Metabolism, Johns Hopkins University, 1830 East Monument Street, Suite 328, Baltimore, MD 21287
e-mail: adobs@jhmi.edu

is difficult, developing integrative services within an academic medical center can provide patients with more options and greater comfort.

Keywords: Johns Hopkins · Complementary And Integrative Medicine · program development · challenges · acupuncture · massage · mind-body class.

8.1 Introduction

Developing a clinical integrative medical service at Johns Hopkins has been challenging and time consuming. From the start we faced numerous challenges including physician resistance, funding difficulties, and space limitations. This chapter discusses our initial plans, problems and accomplishments in developing a Complementary and Integrative Medicine (CIM) Service within the institution. It is meant as a guide to others on navigating a large academic medical center. Our goal was always to provide our patients with safe and beneficial treatment options. Johns Hopkins has always been known for its commitment to the highest standards of patient care. These attributes were to continue in any new program.

8.2 Clinical Service Initial Stage Development Process

8.2.1 Overview of the Institution

The Johns Hopkins Medical Institution, founded in 1889 in Baltimore, Maryland, consists of several health divisions of Johns Hopkins University, including the School of Medicine, School of Nursing and The Bloomberg School of Public Health. The hospital is situated within an urban east-coast setting.

8.2.2 Early Interest and Planning

In 1999, Catherine De Angelis, MD, Vice Dean for Academic Affairs, convened an open meeting of faculty and staff interested in developing a Complementary and Alternative Medicine (CAM) Research Center. This meeting drew 140 people. It was discovered that there already were 15 ongoing CAM-related research projects in progress. A CAM committee was formed to spearhead the creation of a Johns Hopkins Medicine Center for the Study of CIM. The initial goals were the following:

- Develop a resource to assist Johns Hopkins faculty and staff in the creation of scientifically sound studies involving the use of complementary/integrative modalities.
- Develop an educational resource for patients and providers in complementary/integrative services, including information about defining the modalities,

licensure, certification, safety and efficacy of treatments and sources of care in the community.
- Develop a more scholarly, informed and service oriented response to patients' requests for and use of complementary services. (Catherine DeAngelis' Memo to Dean Miller October 20, 1999)

8.2.3 Creation of a Johns Hopkins Research CAM Center

A Request for Applications for P-50 Center grants was announced by NCCAM in 1999. Dr. Dobs, an established investigator interested in the area, received the support of Dr. DeAngelis to write a grant as Principal Investigator. At this point, Dr. Dobs spent several months identifying potential investigators and core services. The Center grant was focused on cancers, particularly breast and prostate cancer. Key components of the Research Center were four RO1 grants, funds for pilot studies and training opportunities. One of the key features of our program has been a weekly CAM conference open to the entire Hopkins community, in which state of the art lectures, invited speakers and research conferences were presented to broaden the scientific interest in CAM. At a later point, the need for clinical services became evident, resulting in an application and eventual funding from the Kimmel Foundation, a private foundation that had provided funds to the Johns Hopkins Kimmel Oncology Center.

8.2.4 Establish an Advisory Board

Membership on this board was based on interest and was voluntary. Thirty individuals, including physicians, nurses, pharmacists, psychologists, social workers, administrators, pastoral care and dietitians attended the first meeting. They represented the following departments/divisions throughout the medical school: oncology, endocrinology, medicine, psychiatry, pediatrics, dermatology, public health, physical medicine and rehabilitation, gynecology, infectious disease and bioethics. The initial meeting was chaired by the medical director of the department of oncology who emphasized the importance of providing complementary services to our cancer patients.

8.2.5 Search for and Hire a Program Coordinator to Create the Program

We looked for someone who had skills in conventional medicine as well as complementary medicine. We hired an advanced practice nurse/acupuncturist (KM) with the following skills: CAM expertise, program development, administration, healthcare reimbursement, marketing and public speaking. This is one model, that is, choosing a nurse who had expertise in both conventional medicine and integrative therapies. However, another approach could have been used, that is, hiring an individual with more administrative skill who would be responsible for setting up a program and hiring/expanding services by bringing on specific CAM expertise. This decision could be based on resources and availability of CAM personnel.

8.3 Practical Aspects in Planning a Complementary and Integrative Medicine Service

8.3.1 Establish a Steering Committee

This committee consisted of the medical director of the CAM research program (Dr. Dobs), the oncology administrator/director of oncology nursing, the director of patient care services and the new nurse program coordinator (K. Menten). This committee was responsible for the orientation of the new program coordinator and the creation of the general direction of the new service. In addition, this committee was responsible for the creation of the mission statement and philosophy of the Complementary and Integrative Service.

8.3.2 Survey Other Institutions

We made site visits to two neighboring institutions to better understand their services, challenges and funding issues. They helped us to avoid some of the pitfalls in creating a new program. In addition, they provided us with a wealth of information regarding where we need to place the most focus. We are grateful that these institutions were willing to share information with us.

8.3.3 Survey Current Hopkins Employees to Identify Qualified CAM Practitioners

Johns Hopkins is the largest employer in the State of Maryland, employing over 24,000 people. We tried to identify Hopkins employees with certification and experience to provide services. They would be familiar with the Hopkins' system and facilitate any hiring procedures. Although we had approximately five acupuncturists already on staff, most of them were foreign trained and unable to obtain a Maryland License. We were more fortunate in the massage arena. Several of our oncology nurses were also certified massage therapists, who were acutely aware of the medical needs of oncology patients. They were instrumental in the formulation of massage policies, procedures and job descriptions. We gave hiring preference to oncology nurses who are also massage therapists or acupuncturists.

8.3.4 Conduct Administrative Meetings with Representatives from Key Departments

To ensure support from a wide range of administrative functions, we met with oncology administration, medicine, nursing, legal departments, human resources, finance, billing, medical records, credentialing and public affairs. These meetings laid the foundation and established the ground rules for the development of our new service. The types of services to be developed were new and different to the institution. These meetings were often highly charged as people presented opposite points of view. For example, CAM services provided in the community are usually paid directly by the patient. This model is rarely applied in a large academic medical center, where the majority of patients have some form of insurance. There were long hours of discussion around the ethics of providing services to only a minority of patients able to afford out-of-pocket expenses.

8.3.5 Key Issues Discussed in the Initial Planning Stages

What patient population is to be served? Initially, we decided to serve the outpatient population in oncology only. Soon requests came to treat inpatients. After careful consideration, we agreed to provide services to inpatients. It also solved the problem of where to provide services in an institution that has outgrown its' designated space.

What is the risk/benefit ratios for proposed services? It was decided to offer acupuncture, massage and mind-body classes as first steps. Acupuncture and massage are both licensed in the State of Maryland. Another advantage of acupuncture was that a national board certification process was already in place (NCCAOM, National Certification Commission for Acupuncture and Oriental Medicine). Because we require board certification of our physicians, we decided to also require it of our acupuncturists. Our latest service is the integrative medicine consult. One of our holistic MD's will be responsible for these.

Who should provide the services—outside providers versus hospital employee? Contractual providers were initially not allowed by the legal department, due to malpractice issues. However, that was later changed and massage is now offered by an independent contractor who is bound by Hopkins' policies, procedures, protocols and job descriptions.

Moonlighting providers? This issue is currently being discussed. We have had residents and fellows who are also medical acupuncturists request to moonlight on our service. The issues that have arisen are focused on whether they can be supervised by another medical acupuncturist who is an attending physician, because they are considered trainees here. If we contract with providers, are job descriptions needed? Yes, we are ultimately legally responsible for the performance of these practitioners. Therefore, we needed to write job descriptions, procedures, protocols and so on.

Are MD referrals necessary for provision of these services? We decided insist upon MD referrals for several reasons: (1) we would be more likely to get third party reimbursement, (2) we wanted the doctors aware of and in agreement with their patients obtaining acupuncture and massage and (3) we wanted to encourage communication between the physicians and the complementary medicine practitioners in order to provide a truly integrative service.

Are standards of care, protocols, policies, procedures necessary for all of the CAM services provided? We developed policies and procedures for all offerings. It is our way of assuring that the excellent quality of care that is present everywhere else in this institution is adhered to in these services.

How should we credential these practitioners? It was decided that acupuncturists should be credentialed as affiliate medical staff and that the medical staff credentialing department should be responsible for this process. Massage therapists would be credentialed by the program coordinator for complementary medicine. Once it was decided to contract out for massage services, the owner of the business supplying massage was held responsible for the credentialing process.

What are the documentation requirements for these practitioners? Acupuncturists are required to dictate into the electronic patient record. They are required to use the same format as physicians do, adding information pertinent to acupuncture. The program coordinator created a "cheat sheet" for acupuncturists, which allows them to take notes in the same order and format as the required dictation. Massage therapists will use a form that goes on what is left of our paper chart. Once we move to an exclusively electronic chart, this form will be filled out electronically. Ultimately we decided to offer a one hour drop and relaxations guided imagery class. This has been well received.

Table 8.1 Important Questions to be Addressed Before Establishing a Complementary and Integrative Medical (CIM) Service

Questions to address in setting up a CIM Program
Patient population to be served?
Risk/benefit rations for proposed services?
Outside providers versus employee providers?
Moonlighting providers?
Are MD referrals necessary? If so, for which services?
Are standards of care, policies, procedures, protocols necessary?
How should these practitioners be credentialed?
What are the documentation requirements?

8.4 Services Now Being Provided

8.4.1 Acupuncture

We began our program with acupuncture, a mind-body class and massage. We started with these modalities because they had the advantages of licensure in the State of Maryland, and we already had staff members who were qualified to practice them. Acupuncture also had the advantage of national board certification (NCCAOM). Acupuncture is one component of Traditional Chinese Medicine, a holistic, energy-based approach to healthcare that is more than 2000 years old. It includes a variety of procedures that stimulate specific points on the surface of the body to effect bodily organs and function. This stimulation is achieved through the use of ultra-thin needles, heat, electricity or finger pressure. Acupuncture has been found to be useful for chemotherapy-related nausea and vomiting [1]. In addition, acupuncture's usefulness for the treatment of radiation-induced Xerostomia has been well-documented [2–5]. Although we started acupuncture in the outpatient clinic, we soon began getting referrals for inpatient acupuncture as well.

Table 8.2 Indications for Acupuncture for the Oncology Patient

Indications for acupuncture for the oncology patient
Pain, nociceptive and neuropathic
Nausea
Vomiting
Xerostomia
Neuropathy
Fatigue
Insomnia
Anxiety
Depression
Other symptom control as needed

Table 8.3 Contraindications for Acupuncture for the Oncology Patient [8, 9]

General Contraindications	**Additional electro-acupuncture contraindications**
Acute cardiac arrhythmias	Pacemaker
Lymphedema (no needles in affected limb)	History of heart disease
Cancerous growths (no needles in or near)	Seizure disorder
Skin lesions (no needles in local area)	Lack of skin sensation
Severely disturbed patients	
Lab values: WBC <1500 #/CU MM	
ANC <500 #/cu mm	
Platelet count <50 K/CU MM	
Forbidden points	
Semi-permanent needle contraindications	**Precautions**
Valvular heart disease	Extremely fatigued patients
Neutropenic patients (ANC <500 cu mm)	Anticoagulant use (discuss INR level with MD)
Post-splenectomy patients	Immunodeficiency (WBC >3000 use sterile technique)
Known hepatitis	Impaired sensation
During cycles of chemotherapy and radiation	Pregnancy
	Unstable diabetes
	Hungry patients

8.4.2 Massage Therapy

Massage is defined as using one's hands to apply pressure and motion on the skin and underlying muscle of the recipient for the purposes of physical and psychological relaxation, improvement of circulation, relief of sore muscles and other therapeutic benefits. Our high-tech interventions for patient care have the disadvantage of only touching the patient for a procedure that is usually painful. Long gone are the days when nurses gave patients backrubs. This is indeed unfortunate, especially for patients who are in the hospital for longer stays. Touch conveys a sense of warmth, caring, security and comfort, in addition to the benefits of massage described above.

Table 8.4 Indications for Massage Therapy in Oncology Patients

Indications for massage in oncology patients [10, 11]
Musculoskeletal discomfort due to taught, tense muscles and tendons
Pain
Lymphedema (special training and certification required)
Mental stress, tension and fatigue
Insomnia
Anxiety
Need for touch

Table 8.5 Contraindications for Massage in Oncology Patients

Contraindications for Massage in Oncology Patients [10, 11]	
Contraindications	**Areas to avoid massage**
Fever	Directly on tumor site
Hemophilia	Directly over radiation sites
Abdominal aneurysm	Over swollen joints
Sepsis	Over varicose veins
Thrombosis or DVT	Fracture site
Multiple myeloma	Phlebitis
Bone fragility, unstable spine	Cellutis
Radioactive implants	Rash/ open wounds
Long-term steroid use	Burns/ damaged skin
Use of: anticoagulant or thrombolytic drugs	Pacemaker boxes
Labs: platelet count <10 K/CU MM	IV/VAD sites
Labs: platelet count 10–50 K comfort touch massage only; requires MD order	Implantable device sites
Labs: WBC <1000 comfort touch massage only, requires MD order	Transdermal patch sites
Precautions	
Osteoporosis	
Pleural effusion	
History of myoglobulinemia	

8.4.3 Mind-Body Class

The mind-body class we chose for patients was benchmarked on Jon Kabet-Zinn's Mindfulness-Based Stress Reduction. It is a 6-week, 12-h class that covers topics like relaxation, guided imagery, mindfulness meditation, belly breathing, stress reduction, coping skills, managing side effects, addressing grief, fear and loss and creating new possibilities. This class has not been well accepted or sought out by patients, even though our nursing staff have been very enthusiastic about it. More thought needs to go why patients have resisted this. Physicians have reported in our pain conference that they have suggested the class to patients and handed them a brochure, yet they do not call. The 6-week commitment may be an issue, along with the fact that we need to charge for this class in order to provide it.

8.4.4 Integrative Medicine Consult Service

An Integrative Medicine Consultation is a patient-centered evaluation by a holistic physician consisting of a detailed review of the patient's medical history and medical record. This includes medications, herbs and supplements taken (or patient's questions about taking).Other things to be considered are nutrition, lifestyle, stressors, and conventional and non-conventional treatments. Both traditional and non-traditional diagnostic tests may be recommended. Once all of this in formation is compiled, recommendations are made for a range of therapeutic interventions from both conventional and complementary medicine. These may include diet, medications, herbs, supplements and various interventions for body (massage, acupuncture), mind (mind-body class) and spirit (meditation).

8.5 Administration of the CIM Service

8.5.1 Credentialing

Joint Commission on Accreditation for Hospitals requires that anyone having therapeutic contact with patients be credentialed. At first our credentialing office was reluctant to consider the credentialing of non-physician acupuncturists as affiliate medical staff. However, when they were presented with the educational requirements for becoming an acupuncturist (over 2000 hours) and the requirements for the accreditation of acupuncture schools, they changed their minds.

The credentialing department asked our help in writing the credentialing piece for acupuncture, including the delineation of privileges. Once written, this was taken to the credentialing committee for final acceptance. We required 5 years of experience and NCCAOM board certification of acupuncturists. Inpatient work with patients at the complexity level we have here at Johns Hopkins requires that a person be very well grounded in the practice of acupuncture as well as the principles of treatment. Although acupuncture was to be provided only in oncology initially, the credentialing packet was created to serve the entire institution. It has taken 9 months for our first acupuncturist to be approved.

Indications for treatment include acute and chronic pain control, addiction control, cancer-related symptoms, circulatory disorders, dermatological disorders, eye, ear, nose and throat disorders, emotional and psychological disorders, gastrointestinal disorders, gynecological/ genitourinary disorders, immune disorders/autoimmune disorders, neurological disorders, respiratory disorders and palliative care. We used the World Health Organization's list of disorders that acupuncture has been found to help as our basis for this list [6].

8.5.2 Policies/Procedures

Our goals were to provide the structure and outline the parameters under which acupuncture could be practiced here at Johns Hopkins. Unfortunately, there were no publications listing laboratory precautions for acupuncture. After discussions with comparable institutions, MD Anderson and Memorial Sloan Kettering, we positioned ourselves somewhere in between, that is, patients need to have the following counts to qualify for acupuncture: platelets 50 K/CU MM, ANC 500 CU MM, and WBC 1500 CU MM. We have had no problems working within these parameters. In addition, as acupuncture punctures the skin, we required approval from our infection control committee. We established the techniques as described in the *Clean Needle Technique Manual for Acupuncturists* [7].

8.5.3 Job Descriptions

Formal job descriptions were created. They described scope of responsibility, decision making, authority, communication channels, education requirements, experience, certification, licensure, credentialing, physical requirements and supervision. We have written job descriptions for the program coordinator, acupuncturists and massage therapists. The massage therapist who works for our independent contractor must adhere to our job description requirements.

8.5.4 Developing Clinical Forms

The development of intake, consent to treat and discharge forms for acupuncture was very time consuming. Our legal department demanded that we provide them with the exact percentages of every known side effect and adverse effect for acupuncture. Once the numbers were compiled, our lawyers then decided which one's needed to be on the consent form. After the legal department made their final decision, the forms then went to our forms committee for finalization. This entire process took several months. The massage forms did not have to go through the legal department, however, they did have to go through our forms committee because they were to become part of the medical record.

8.5.5 Liaisons

We appreciated the need to create liaisons with a wide range of hospital personnel. There are numerous competing demands on departments and often a CIM Service is a low priority. It is much easier to move your agenda through a committee by working closely with other departments. The time it takes to establish and nurture these relationships is very well spent. Once the program is up and running, there will be many times that things need to be changed or added. These liaisons are invaluable in both the creation and the ongoing maintenance of a program. Establishing a good rapport with several physicians is also very necessary to keep patients flowing into the program.

8.6 Financial Aspects

8.6.1 Negotiating Billing Procedures

Billing procedures dictated how we would hire acupuncturists and massage therapists. Both had to be considered "pro-fee" providers. That automatically meant that these practitioners had to be employed by the university rather than the hospital. It gets very confusing when both university and hospital employees work side by side in the hospital. Before hiring anyone, make sure that you are aware of the policies in your institution.

Billing has been a major problem for us. For the first year, we billed patients' insurance, thus requiring that our acupuncturist became a provider for each insurance company with whom Johns Hopkins had a contractual relationship. This took several months. Next, the billing office needed to be appraised of the CPT codes for acupuncture and a dollar amount had to be assigned to each code. It was decided to use a paper voucher, rather than deal with our electronic billing system. We were not allowed to collect any monies up front, rather the insurance company was billed, and only after they paid were we allowed to bill patients. Consequently, our income was severely limited. Now we "opt out" of all insurance and require that acupuncture patients pay up front and then get reimbursed later. This is a model that most patients are already used to, because most acupuncturists operate this way.

8.6.2 Space

Space is at a very high premium everywhere on our medical campus. It was thought to be very important to offer CIM services in the same outpatient area as the rest of our other outpatient services. As a result we negotiated for, and received, one room in the oncology outpatient center for half a day twice per week. At this point, we are not required to pay rent, the usual practice in our institution. The administration in oncology recognized that it would be impossible for the new service to pay rent for this room. Massage will be offered in an office near the Radiation Oncology offices.

Although we also wanted to have a presence at our more suburban center, the rent there made it a financial impossibility. Fortunately, Johns Hopkins is building a new family and patient care center which will be located across the street from our oncology center. We have reserved two dedicated rooms in that new building which is projected to be completed in 2 years.

8.6.3 Equipment

Fortunately, acupuncture requires very little equipment. We ordered sterile, disposable acupuncture needles of various sizes, sterile towels and gloves, and two small electro-acupuncture devices. Because we are dealing with patients whose immune systems are compromised, we decided to use chlorohexidine preps rather than alcohol preps. Space blankets make great covers for acupuncture patients because they are so light and fluffy.

We bought massage tables that were longer, wider and softer than average in order to provide more comfort for patients who are already in pain. Acupuncture works better when patients are able to be completely relaxed during the session. The tables also had a built in back rest for patients who needed to be in an upright position for treatment. These were initially set up and taken down in an exam room before and after each scheduled acupuncture morning in the outpatient clinic. This was very labor and time intensive, so we eventually bought a table that could also be used as an exam table.

8.6.4 Scheduling

We decided to take advantage of an already existing scheduling service in the outpatient department of oncology for acupuncture. In order to do this, new forms needed to be created, new policies for how to schedule were created and several in-service education sessions were held with the schedulers and financial counselors to briefly explain the concepts of acupuncture and outline the process through which patients would get scheduled for this service.

8.6.5 Referrals

In order to facilitate communication with our physicians and provide easy ways for them to refer a patient, the medical director and program coordinator introduced the CIM Service at a faculty meeting. We distributed a laminated referral card that would fit in the pockets of the standard white medical coat. This card included indications and contraindications for acupuncture, as well as the eligibility criteria for patients. Similar meetings occurred with the oncology fellows to introduce the CIM service.

8.6.6 Marketing

Once a program is developed, marketing becomes extremely important. Determining the target market is the first priority. Due to our extremely limited space, we determined that we would start with current oncology patients in our center. If they did not fill the time slots allotted, then we would branch out. We have not needed to branch out. Our greatest problem is finding more space.

We created brochures for the mind-body class and for acupuncture. The brochures were distributed to staff in all of the in-service education offerings, placed in every treatment and consultation room, and made available in the main waiting rooms for medical and radiation oncology. In addition, we created large, color posters that were placed in the waiting rooms of the oncology clinics.

Our marketing efforts were concentrated within our medical system. The program coordinator scheduled separate in-service education sessions for the nursing staff, the medical oncology fellows, the radiation oncology fellows, social workers and the cancer pain interdisciplinary team. There were separate sessions on acupuncture and on the mind-body classes we intended to offer. At first, they resulted in very few referrals. Because CAM is a patient-driven initiative, we also did marketing directly to patients with the brochures and posters. Many patients have called after seeing the acupuncture poster in the waiting rooms. The mind-body class has not had enough patient interest to warrant starting it.

Johns Hopkins has many internal communication newsletters and magazines. We took advantage of all of them over the period of 1 year. In addition, we took advantage of the local newspapers that were willing to report that we had started a complementary medicine service.

8.7 Education Programs

Even before the program was completed, there was a tremendous upsurge of interest in various aspects of CAM. Health care providers appreciate the need to understand CAM to better inform and make recommendations to their patients. Scientists are beginning to see the immense need for research in the field. Our educational programming includes (1) weekly scientific presentations on research, (2) state-of-the art in-service education offerings on acupuncture and mind-body education to nursing staff, (3) Institutional CME conferences, for example, palliative care, cancer pain, breast cancer, and a two-day CAM CME conference, and (4) lay programs, for example, Woman's Journey Conference and the National Breast Cancer Coalition Conference. We believe that building a service requires a familiarity with the services and science behind it. The program coordinators, as well as the medical director, were involved with teaching groups of health care providers throughout the medical center.

8.8 Case Study

As an example of our work, we present a patient who was seen in consultation by the CIM service. This case illustrates the effectiveness of acupuncture in helping to maintain some comfort and quality of life in a seriously ill patient who was in end stage disease.

Mr. F. was a 45-year-old Caucasian male who had been hospitalized 3 months earlier for evaluation of an esophageal-gastric junction mass diagnosed as metastatic esophageal adenocarcinoma with metastasis to the stomach and liver. He had progressed through two cycles of chemotherapy, during which time he developed intractable hiccups, nausea, vomiting and subsequent weight loss. In addition, he was suffering from pulmonary atelectasis and mild depression in adjusting to the seriousness of this illness. His physician called the acupuncture service to see if anything could be done to help this man's intractable hiccups. Lastly, the patient wanted treatment for pain in his lower back, insomnia, fatigue, depression and anxiety.

On history, review of systems and physical examination was noteworthy for: tachycardia, shortness of breath with retractions, intractable hiccups, severe diarrhea, esophageal pain, nausea, vomiting, concentrated amber colored urine, lumbosacral back pain (VAS 3), insomnia, depression, anxiety and fearfulness. In addition he had a central IV port in his upper right chest and a peripheral IV in his left forearm. He was NPO.

From a Traditional Chinese Medicine standpoint, his tongue was narrow with a red body and a very thick, wet, greasy coat and a deep center crack with a very red tip. His energetic pulses were thin, wiry and fast with the first position pulses on both wrists barely palpable and the middle position on both wrists very excess. The Chinese diagnosis was a combination of damp heat in the middle burner, stomach and liver blood stasis, lung and spleen chi deficiency, rebellious stomach chi and heart fire.

Mr. F. seemed desperate to obtain some relief. The initial intervention was to teach him how to stimulate the acupuncture point conception vessel 22. Once he learned this, he was able to control the hiccups, providing that he intervened early enough. He was so pleased with this particular intervention that he called his physicians back to show them his newly acquired skill. He was then needled, and during the procedure while the needles were being retained, he was being taught deep, belly breathing as the needles were being manipulated. His breathing improved immediately and his hiccups had already stopped. He was so pleased that he asked for and received daily acupuncture treatments. The acupuncturist was asked to join daily rounds to report on and explain what they were doing to the treating interdisciplinary team. A truly integrative process ensued in which meaningful dialog occurred.

Unfortunately, Mr. F. was in the end stage of his illness and his prognosis was very poor. The acupuncture treatment relaxed him enough that he was able to sleep for hours afterward. His hiccups also decreased significantly. He was very appreciative of this and was eagerly looking forward to his second treatment. His sacral pain had increased to a VAS of 5 and he was still having trouble breathing. After being treated with acupuncture, he was again very relaxed, less anxious and his pain dropped to a VAS of 1.

Four days passed between treatment number 3 and 4. Mr. F's condition was rapidly deteriorating. His main complaint was breathlessness. His respirations were quite labored with sternal retractions and nasal flaring, despite being on Oxygen. He was extremely anxious about this. In addition he remained tachycardic. New symptoms that presented themselves were scrotal swelling which was extremely uncomfortable, dependent edema, mottled legs and bluish-black soles of his feet. The nausea and vomiting were gone. His back pain was under control with the use of a lidocaine patch. Clearly, the priority was breathing and supporting his entire system, which was beginning to shut down. After an acupuncture treatment, his breathing improved noticeably while the needles were retained.

Mr. F. deteriorated further overnight. When the acupuncturist arrived the next morning, he had his head thrown back and was gasping with agonal breathing, wheezing, nasal flaring and retractions in the neck, chest and abdominal area. He was sweating profusely and his skin had a greenish cast to it. There was pitting, dependent edema and scrotal swelling. He was extremely anxious. The acupuncturist focused on points that would help restore breathing. His response to this acupuncture treatment was truly remarkable. Thirty seconds after the needles were inserted, he stopped sweating, stopped gasping for breath and turned to the acupuncturist saying, "thank you, I can breathe." The acupuncturist proceeded to ask his attending physician if she could leave ear tacks on the lung points for better lung functioning, explaining that this might help his breathless feeling and give him some sense of control over his deteriorating situation. Ear tacks were place on the lung points in Mr. F's ears and his wife was instructed in the care of these points as well as on the use of acupressure points for his lungs. He was discharged to home hospice the next morning.

8.9 Challenges Faced by the Complementary and Integrative Medicine Service

We see several ongoing challenges to the continued growth of a CIM Service. The Johns Hopkins Medical Institutions has a reputation for providing world class conventional, evidence-based medicine. The medical community is unclear on the role and efficacy of acupuncture and other CAM modalities. This hurdle will require more rigorous research in the field, as well as education the physician on the theories and practice of CAM.

There is also resistance from our patients. They often come to our institution expecting the success of conventional medicine. Some physicians question whether they will be accepting of our use of treatments that may not have a strong evidence base. Patients need to understand that many of the commonly used therapies are themselves unproven. In addition, we need to emphasize to our patients that CAM clinical offerings are not to treat the underlying condition, as much as to improve quality of life.

A third challenge facing our growth is reimbursement for procedures. Our medical care system is an insurance-based system. Patients coming to the hospital do not expect to pay out of pocket, but rather demand that insurance pay. The reimbursement was so low that we have now chosen to opt out of insurance coverage. The possibility of financial profit or even covering costs is unlikely within a large academic medical center. Philanthropic support appears to be a necessity. Perhaps, our biggest impediment at this juncture is the lack of adequate space to provide services. Conventional forms of treatment take precedence and are given priority.

8.10 Conclusions/Summary

CIM has an important role in hospitals and outpatient clinics. It provides the patients with procedures that address quality of life issues while they are receiving conventional treatments that may make them very uncomfortable. Providing these services under the auspices of the hospital helps patients feel more comfortable about the safety and efficacy of the treatments provided. It also provides patients with choices when conventional treatment is painful or ineffective with a poor prognosis.

In this chapter, we described the essential steps needed for the planning, development and implementation of a CIM Service within Johns Hopkins Medical System. Multi-department and multidisciplinary planning and cooperation is of utmost importance in the creation of such a service. The service must comply with the existing organizational parameters of the institution.

Initial stages require a multidisciplinary planning process that addresses the following issues: patient population, employed practitioners versus independent contractors, risk/benefit ratio for services, standards of care, policies and procedures, referral requirements, and documentation requirements, credentialing, billing and form development.

The establishment and nurturing of liaisons in each department is critical to the success of the program. Marketing is also an important factor in the success of the program. The right people need to know about your services to utilize them. Patients need to be made aware of services available as they will take the initiative and do what is necessary to receive them. Professional and patient education enables the faculty, staff and patients to understand the advantages and the dangers of various CAM modalities.

The greatest challenge of maintaining these programs is the financial aspect. The reimbursement level is complicated and insufficient to building a program. Endowment or some philanthropic support is necessary to offset the cost of running a Complementary and Integrative Program.

Acknowledgments Portion of this manuscript has been supported by the Kimmel Foundation in the Johns Hopkins Kimmel Oncology Center.

References

1. NIH. Acupuncture. NIH Consensus Statement. 1997; Nov. 3–5; 15(5):1–34.
2. Johnstone PAS, Peng YP, May BC, Inouye WS, Niemzow RC. Acupuncture for pilocarpine-resistant xerostomia following radiotherapy for head and neck malignancies. Int J Radiat Oncol Biol Phys 2001; 50(2):353–7.
3. Blom M, Dawidson I, Angmar-Mansson B. The effect of acupuncture on salivary flow rates in patients with xerostomia. Oral Surg Oral Med Oral Pathol 1992; 73:293–8.
4. Johnstone PAS, Niemzow RC, Rittenburgh RH. Acupuncture for Xerostomia clinical update. Cancer 2002; 94(4):1151–6.
5. Wong RK, Jones GW, Sagar SM, Angelica-Fargus B, Whelan T. A Phase I-II study in the use of acupuncture-like transcutaneous nerve stimulation in the treatment of radiation-induced xerostomia in head and neck cancer patients treated with radical radiotherapy. Int J Radiat Oncol Biol Phys 2003; 57(2):472–80.
6. Lee BY, LaRiccia PJ, Newberg AB. Acupuncture in Theory and Practice Part 2: Clinical Indications, Efficacy and Safety. World Health Organization (WHO) Interregional Seminar, June 1979. Hospital Physician. 2004; 40(5):33–38.
7. Clean Needle Technique Manual for Acupuncturists. Fifth edition, National Acupuncture Foundation, 2003.
8. Acupuncture Policy. West Lincolnshire NHS 2004–2005.
9. MacPherson H, Thomas K, Walters S, Fitter M. A prospective survey of adverse events and treatment reactions following 34,000 consultations with professional acupuncturists. Acupuncture in Medicine. 2001 Dec; 19(2):93–102.
10. White A, Hayhoe S, Hart A, Ernst E; BMAS and AACP. British Medical Acupuncture Society and Acupuncture Association of Chartered Physiotherapists. Survey of adverse events follwoing acupuncture (SAFA): a prospective study of 32,000 consultations. Acupuncture in Medicine. 2001 Dec; 19(2):84–92.
11. Gecsedi, RA. Massage Therapy for patients with cancer. Clinical Journal of Oncology Nursing 2002; 6(1):52–4.

Chapter 9
Integrative Oncology at Mayo Clinic

Research Informing Practice

Debra L. Barton, Brent A. Bauer and Charles L. Loprinzi

Contents

9.1	Research in Integrative Medicine and Oncology	124
9.2	Research Summary	131
9.3	Conclusion	134
References		134

Abstract The role of research has been integrally tied to the primary goal of patient care as well as education, consistent with Mayo Clinic's philosophy that medicine must be developed as a cooperative science between the clinician, the specialist, and the laboratory, all for the good of the patient. This chapter reviews Mayo Clinic's experience with studying and implementing complementary therapy interventions for patients as well as the integration of education to the broader staff and public about various CAM modalities. In 2002, because of continuing interest from patients in Complementary and Alternative Medicine (CAM) treatments, a collaborative team was created to investigate CAM modalities being utilized by cancer patients. The ultimate goal of this team was to bring reliable scientific evidence to practice so that both patients and physicians could make informed decisions about the various treatments and modalities. The Mayo Complementary and Integrative Medicine Program and Division of Medical Oncology clinicians and researchers have been partnering to expand the evidence base in CAM in order to expand treatment options for patients. Clinical trials developed and implemented in both symptom management and treatment for cancer are discussed. In addition, the application of the research findings to education and clinical practice is described. A monthly seminar series was created to provide a forum for dissemination of the research findings. A review of topics is included. The Integrative Medicine Consult Service was established in 2004, and various services and care options for patients are discussed, as well as the inclusion of data regarding patient referrals.

B.A. Bauer
Director, Complementary and Integrative Medicine Program, Mayo Clinic, 200 1st St SW, Rochester, MN 55905
e-mail: bauer.brent@mayo.edu

Keywords: Integrative medicine · research · education · patient care.

The Mayo Clinic Cancer Center, from its inception, has adhered to the Mayo Clinic primary value, "The needs of the patient come first". This has been evidenced by the fact that the Mayo Clinic Cancer center was one of the first National Cancer Institute designated comprehensive cancer centers, with over 16,000 new patients treated each year.

The role of research has been integrally tied to the care patient as well as education, consistent with Mayo Clinic's philosophy that medicine must be developed as a cooperative science between the clinician, the specialist and the laboratory, all for the good of the patient.

In 2002, because of continuing interest from patients in Complementary and Alternative Medicine (CAM) treatments, a collaborative team was created to investigate in a scientifically rigorous fashion, CAM modalities being utilized by cancer patients. The goal of this team was to bring reliable scientific evidence to practice so that both patients and physicians could make informed decisions about the various treatments and modalities.

One of the partners in this research endeavor has been the Complementary and Integrative Medicine Program at the Mayo Clinic, which was founded in July 2001 as a program within the Department of Medicine (DOM). This Program was created to help address the ever increasing patient interest in wellness-promoting activities which are not typically part of conventional medical care. The program incorporates the three prongs of Mayo Clinic's philosophy and provides a framework for the partnering of research, education and patient care.

To date, the popular use of complementary therapies has mostly preceded their evidence base. However, as research about these therapies is growing, it is increasingly possible to identify those therapies that may have potential benefit, are safe and can be integrated into the total approach to healthcare. Combining the best of conventional medicine with the best evidence-based therapies from the complementary realm has yielded the concept of "Integrative Medicine". It is this emerging integration of the best of all possible practices that informs the vision of the Mayo Complementary and Integrative Medicine Program today. The specific vision of this Complementary and Integrative Medicine Program is twofold. First, it is to continually discover and study, in a collaborative fashion, the expanding realm of Integrative Medicine and second to share and employ that knowledge to ensure Mayo Clinic continues to provide the most complete care of our patients: body, mind and spirit.

9.1 Research in Integrative Medicine and Oncology

Many institutions are implementing integrative medicine clinics to provide patients the option of combining complementary therapies with standard, conventional medical care. In this era of evidence-based medicine, it is important that integrative medicine clinics incorporate and promote practices that have been studied in rigorously designed trials and have been proven to be helpful. To promote interventions without good evidence of efficacy is to waste resources in terms of time, toxicity and often money as complementary interventions are not cost-free. Therefore, one barrier that might be encountered by centers attempting to offer integrative clinics is a dearth of published, well-designed trials that can inform providers and patients about the risks and benefits of various complementary treatments.

At the Mayo Clinic, we have used our various research venues to try to compensate for the paucity of evidence by developing and completing studies with popular complementary interventions that had minimal to no published evidence base. This has been true related to both symptom management and for treatment of cancer.

Investigators at the Mayo Clinic have completed 19 clinical trials regarding complementary therapies and have published these in peer reviewed clinical journals. Four other trials have been completed and are in press or being analyzed, and four trials are actively accruing patients, with two of these close to completing accrual requirements. Phase III clinical trials have involved a number of areas of symptom management and cancer treatment, including hot flash management, anorexia/cachexia, mucosal injury and skin reactions, and treatment for advanced cancer. Most of these phase III clinical trials in oncology symptom management have been done in the large, cooperative setting of the North Central Cancer Treatment Group (NCCTG) involving over 30 community cancer centers. The Mayo Clinic serves as the research base for this group. The full list of completed and published studies is listed in Table 9.1. Experience with research in a few key areas will be reviewed.

9.1.1 Hot Flashes

Menopausal symptoms, in particular hot flashes, are prevalent symptoms that prompt women to seek alternative treatments. In a study by Harris [1], breast cancer survivors were 5.3 times more likely to experience menopausal symptoms and 7.4 times more likely to use alternative treatments, such as herbal remedies, than matched women in the general population. Therefore, efforts at the Mayo Comprehensive Cancer Center as well as internal medicine colleagues have set about to evaluate several popular herbal and dietary supplements used for hot flashes. These have included vitamin E, soy, black cohosh, dehydroepiandrosterone (DHEA) and acupuncture.

9.1.1.1 Vitamin E

Vitamin E had been written about in women's health reference books as an effective intervention for hot flashes, but it had never been formally studied. Therefore, we conducted a placebo-controlled randomized double-blind trial involving 120 women who received either a placebo or active vitamin E, 400 IU twice per day for 4 weeks, and then were crossed over to the opposite treatment for 4 weeks [2]. The outcome measure was a prospective, self-report hot flash daily diary. Patients

Table 9.1 Complementary and Alternative Medicine Studies and Status

Symptom/Toxicity	Agent	Number of patients	Journal, year
Mucosal/epidermal	Cryotherapy	95	JCO, 1991 (18)
Mucosal/epidermal	Cryotherapy duration	178	Cancer, 1993 (19)
Mucosal/epidermal	Chamomile mouthwash	164	Cancer, 1996 (20)
Mucosal/epidermal	Ocular cryotherapy	38	Cancer, 1994 (21)
Mucosal/epidermal	Capsaicin lozenge	18	Journal of Cancer Integrative Medicine, 2004 (22)
Mucosal/epidermal	Aloe vera gel	194	Int J Rad Onc Biol Phys 1996 (23)
Hot flashes	Vitamin E	105	JCO, 1998 5(2)
Hot flashes	Soy	149	JCO, 2000 (3)
Hot flashes	Black cohosh	21	Cancer Investigation, 2004 (4)
Hot flashes	Black cohosh	116	JCO, in press (5)
Hot flashes	DHEA	22	Supportive Cancer Therapy, 2006 (7)
Hot flashes	Acupuncture	103	Menopause, in press (8)
Pain	Capsaicin cream	99	JCO, 1997 (9)
Lymphedema	Coumarin	130	NEJM, 1999 (24)
Anorexia/cachexia colorectal cancer	Hydrazine sulfate	127	JCO, 1994 (10)
Anorexia/cachexia non-small cell lung cancer	Hydrazine sulfate	237	JCO, 1997 (11)
Anorexia/cachexia	Eicosapentaenoic acid	421	JCO, 2004 (12)
Treatment	Laetrile	178	NEJM, 1982 (13)
Treatment	Vitamin C	123	NEJM, 1979 (14)
Treatment	Green tea	42	Cancer, 2003 (15)
Treatment	Shark cartilage	83	Cancer, 2005 (17)

receiving vitamin E had approximately a 50% reduction in hot flashes. However, this was only one less hot flash per day than was experienced by patients receiving the placebo [2], so, although vitamin E was statistically significantly better than was placebo, the clinical significance was not very impressive.

9.1.1.2 Soy Phytoestrogens

Soy phytoestrogens represent another popular hot flash remedy, based in part, on the belief that Asian populations have a diet rich in soy and do not seem to experience hot flashes to the same degree as do women in the Western culture. A randomized, double-blind, placebo-controlled, crossover trial was designed to study the effects of soy on hot flashes [3]. Women were randomized to get 150 mg of isoflavones per day, taken in three divided doses, or an identical-appearing placebo, three times per day. The self-report daily hot flash diary was again used as the primary outcome measure. Evaluable data were available on 149 patients. Soy isoflavones were no more effective at reducing hot flashes than was the placebo [3]. In fact, more patients on the placebo arm reported a 50% reduction in their hot flashes than on the soy isoflavone arm. There were no differences in toxicity between the two groups.

9.1.1.3 Black Cohosh

Black cohosh is another widely used herb for hot flashes. Two studies at the Mayo Clinic have been completed evaluating black cohosh for hot flashes. One was a pilot study [4] and the second, a larger, double-blind, randomized, placebo-controlled trial [5]. The initial pilot trial, involving 23 patients, showed an encouraging reduction in hot flashes with no suggestions of adverse events [4]. Based on these data, a subsequent placebo-controlled trial was developed and completed. This more definitive study, with 116 women, showed that hot flash reductions were more substantial in patients receiving the placebos, than in the patients receiving black cohosh [5].

The placebo effect for hot flashes is known to be about 20–25% [6]. Despite this, agents tested in pilot trials that reduce hot flashes by more than 50% are expected to be effective when tested in larger placebo-controlled trials. Interestingly, though black cohosh reduced hot flash frequency by 51% and hot flash score by 57% in the open-label pilot trial, it only reduced hot flash score by 20% in the placebo-controlled trial. This experience reconfirms that we need to be critical of phase II data and should be careful to not base treatment decisions on incomplete evidence.

9.1.1.4 Dhea

DHEA is a nutritional supplement that is an inactive prohormone, endogenously produced by the adrenal gland and liver. It is converted peripherally to testosterone and estrodiol. The androgenic activity of DHEA provides the rationale for studying this agent in alleviating hot flashes. A pilot study with 22 evaluable women was conducted, and a median hot flash score reduction of 64% from baseline was reported [7]. A larger placebo-controlled dose finding study of DHEA to test the hypothesis that DHEA can reduce hot flashes is currently being developed.

9.1.1.5 Acupuncture

Finally, a study to evaluate acupuncture as a hot flash therapy randomized women to receive either sham or a medical acupuncture with standard points [8]. Results for this study involving 98 patients with evaluable data demonstrated that acupuncture did not significantly reduce hot flashes over the sham intervention [8].

9.1.1.6 Summary

Therefore, based on our program of research, there are currently no dietary supplements that we recommend for our patients to alleviate hot flashes. We are waiting for the larger, more definitive trial on DHEA before deciding whether to incorporate that treatment into our hot flash armamentarium.

9.1.2 Pain

Post-surgical neuropathic pain is another symptom for which there are few effective therapies. Dietary or herbal supplements for pain are popular remedies. One, in particular, capsaicin, a substance made from hot chili peppers, captured the attention of the NCCTG. Chronic neuropathic pain can be a substantial problem for some patients after surgeries such as mastectomy, thoracotomy or limb amputation. This type of pain is often characterized by symptoms of burning, dysthetic numbness and paroxysmal lancinating pain. Capsaicin is known to deplete substance P in small sensory neurons, which is thought to be the mediator of this pain. In this way, it was hypothesized that capsaicin cream could alleviate post-surgical neuropathic pain. A placebo-controlled, double-blind, 8-week crossover study was designed to test the efficacy of capsaicin for post-surgical neuropathic pain [9]. The outcome was evaluated by self-report weekly questionnaires recording pain intensity, pain relief, function deficits related to pain as well as capsaicin related toxicities. The study was completed with 99 evaluable patients and revealed that those patients on capsaicin cream experienced significantly more pain relief. This pain relief was maximized at the end of 4 weeks but was maintained throughout the entire 8 weeks of the study phase. The mean pain reduction on capsaicin was 53%, while the placebo group reported only a 17% mean reduction [9]. Although the toxicities related to the capsaicin cream included a burning sensation on the skin, redness and coughing, overall, the cream was relatively well tolerated. This was evidenced by the fact that there was no difference in the number of patients who stopped treatment on the active agent versus the placebo. The incidence of burning decreased throughout the study period.

9.1.3 Anorexia/Cachexia

Anorexia and cachexia are major issues for many people with advanced cancer, being associated with significant morbidity and mortality. While megestrol acetate (MA) and corticosteroids can ameliorate these problems to a moderate degree, better treatments with a more tolerable side effect profile are needed.

9.1.3.1 Hydrazine Sulfate

Hydrazine sulfate is an organic substance that is a metabolite of isoniazid and is used in industrial processes. Hydrazine sulfate was initially thought to be a potential anticancer agent in the 1970s. It was dropped as an anti-cancer agent by established cancer investigators due to a lack of perceived efficacy, but Dr. Joseph Gold thought hydrazine sulfate could be beneficial for patients with cancer by interrupting cachexia through inhibiting gluconeogenesis. Two studies were undertaken by the Mayo Clinic and the NCCTG to evaluate the role of hydrazine sulfate in advanced cancer [10, 11]. One of the trials accrued patients with advanced colorectal cancer who were resistant to 5FU-based chemotherapy [10]. These patients were randomized to receive 60 mg of hydrazine sulfate versus a placebo, titrating up to two or three capsules per day depending on weight (those weighing more than 50 kg getting three capsules). Participants did not receive active anti-cancer treatment with chemotherapy during this study. The duration of the study intervention was indefinite with the primary endpoint of this trial being survival. With 127 patients evaluated on this study, Kaplan–Meier survival curves revealed no survival advantage for the hydrazine sulfate. In fact, participants receiving hydrazine sulfate had a median survival of 4.3 months, as opposed to 4.7 months for participants on placebo [10]. Quality of life, performance status and weight endpoints were also evaluated. Similar to the survival data, participants on the hydrazine sulfate had more rapidly declining performance status, weight and quality of life, compared to those on placebo, although these were not statistically significant differences [10].

The second trial accrued 237 patients with newly diagnosed non-small cell lung cancer that was not considered to be curable with either surgery or radiation therapy [11]. Hydrazine sulfate 60-mg capsules versus placebo were given with chemotherapy in the same titration schedule as described in the first study. Endpoints included survival and quality of life, the latter measured by the Functional Living Index – Cancer. Neither survival nor quality of life parameters were statistically significantly different between groups, although quality of life parameters tended to be worse in the hydrazine arm [11].

9.1.3.2 Omega 3 Fatty Acids (Eicosapentaenoic Acid)

Omega 3 fatty acids [Eicosapentaenoic acid (EPA)] are dietary supplements believed to have health benefits. Preliminary studies indicated that EPA may have a role in reversing cancer-associated cachexia. Therefore, a double-dummy study design was utilized to test an EPA supplement containing 1.09 g of EPA and 0.46 g of docosahexaenoic acid against MA 600 mg per day versus a combination of both products [12]. Results of this study, which included 421 patients with advanced cancer, revealed that MA was the most effective for weight gain, with 18% of patients gaining 10% over baseline. The EPA arm had 6% of patients achieving a 10% weight gain over baseline. The difference in 10% weight gain between the EPA and MA arm was statistically significantly different ($P = 0.01$).

9.1.3.3 Creatine

Recently, a placebo-controlled clinical trial has been developed and is actively accruing patients to evaluate creatine, an amino acid nutraceutical product used by body builders and other athletes to increase energy, promote muscle mass and enhance athletic performance. Employing a randomized, placebo-controlled, double-blinded study manner, this trial is designed to evaluate whether creatine can help increase weight gain, decrease anorexia and improve quality of life and survival in patients with incurable cancer. The study uses an initial "loading" dose of creatine of 20 g orally per day for 5 days, then decreasing the dose to 2 g per day. Participants will remain on treatment for as long as they perceive benefit.

9.1.3.4 Summary

Again, based on an evaluation of the evidence, there are no dietary supplements or herbal products we currently recommend for anorexia/cachexia in cancer.

9.1.4 Treatment for Advanced Cancer

9.1.4.1 Laetrile

Amygdalin (laetrile), a cyanide containing preparation from apricot pits, was commonly promoted as a promising therapy among non-conventional practitioners in the 1970s. As a result of amygdalin's popularity, Dr. Charles Moertel led a controlled clinical trial with 178 patients with cancer. This trial, published in 1982 in the New England Journal of Medicine, was not able to demonstrate any beneficial effects of laetrile for patients with advanced cancer [13]. Additionally, significant toxicity was identified as the trial revealed blood cyanide levels near the lethal range with the use of amygdalin.

9.1.4.2 Vitamin C

Also in the 1970s, Noble Laureate, Dr. Linus Pauling, claimed that vitamin C was a helpful antidote for patients with cancer. Therefore, many patients commonly took high doses of vitamin C. Again, Dr. Charles Moertel and colleagues prospectively evaluated vitamin C in this setting to provide an evidence base. A study with 123 patients with advanced cancer was completed and published. Participants received oral vitamin C at 10 g per day or a comparably flavored lactose placebo. There was no significant difference in survival between the groups receiving vitamin C versus placebo [14].

9.1.4.3 Green Tea

Green tea has several properties that make it an attractive agent to evaluate as an antineoplastic. New evidence suggests the potential importance of one of its components, epigallocatechin gallate, as an apoptotic agent. Green tea was evaluated by the NCCTG in a phase II trial in men with androgen-independent metastatic prostate cancer [15]. The study used liquid green tea at a dose of 6 g per day in six divided doses. To be eligible, participants' prostate cancers had to be considered to be androgen independent, with rising prostate-specific antigen (PSA) concentrations as the evidence of prostate cancer disease progression. Although men could continue on LHRH (Luteinizing-Hormone-Releasing Hormone) agonists, they could not be on any other treatment for prostate cancer. The primary outcome was the percent of men who sustained a decline in PSA. Forty two patients were studied. Of these, only one patient (2%) had a 50% decrease in PSA levels, but this was not sustained beyond 2 months (15). This 2% response rate was less than the 5% response rate investigators expected to observe due to chance alone.

9.1.4.4 Lycopene

A preliminary investigation of another dietary product, a tomato-based, lycopene-rich product for the treatment of androgen-independent prostate cancer was also completed. Previous studies had designated this carotenoid as a potential cancer preventive agent, and case reports and small, single institution case series suggested antineoplastic effects in patients with malignancies. Based on preliminary evidence, a phase II trial in which all patients received lycopene 30 mg per day in the form of a tomato-based foodstuff was completed. The trial accrued 47 patients, and data analyses are currently ongoing.

9.1.4.5 Shark Cartilage

In the 1990s, the book "Sharks Don't Get Cancer" was the basis for substantial interest in shark cartilage [16]. It was at the height of this interest that the National Cancer Institute requested proposals for randomized, placebo-controlled trials with shark cartilage. Consequently, a study evaluating shark cartilage was developed by the NCCTG, evaluating 96 g per day of shark cartilage versus placebo in patients with advanced breast or colorectal cancer [17]. The recently published results from this trial reported that the shark cartilage was poorly tolerated, with a dropout of 50% of patients within 1 month of study entry [17]. Although designed to accrue 600 patients in order to detect a 33% difference in survival between groups, the study experienced poor accrual and was closed early. The primary endpoint of overall survival was not different between groups for the 83 enrolled subjects, and the quality of life secondary endpoints was also not significantly different between groups.

9.2 Research Summary

Based on the above referenced work, most of the hypothesized dietary or herbal supplement interventions to date that have been rigorously studied by oncology investigators at the Mayo Clinic in Phase III studies have provided negative results and therefore cannot be recommended to be integrated into practice. There are several studies currently accruing patients that have promise, such as ginkgo biloba for chemotherapy-induced cognitive dysfunction, valerian for sleep disturbances and American ginseng for cancer-related fatigue. In addition, positive pilot trials, such as the one with DHEA for hot flashes, will be taken into phase III trials. Research will continue to occur to validate the evidence base for the integration of CAM modalities into standard practice.

9.2.1 Education

Members of the program have a deep commitment to education, both at the professional and public levels. In this regard, colleagues from the Mayo Clinic have delivered over 200 seminars, lectures and talks related to integrative medicine in the past 3 years. These talks have occurred in 15 different states, three different countries and have included national meetings of medical professionals as well as local community groups, women's clubs, church groups and so on. This commitment reflects the dedication of the program leadership to making sure that physicians, patients and consumers have the best information possible to help them make informed decisions about their use of integrative medicine modalities.

A monthly seminar series was created in 2005 and has featured a variety of speakers and topics, such as the following:

- Oriental herbal extracts for prostate cancer prevention and treatment: Discovery of a novel class of anti-androgens, Junxuan Lu, Ph.D, Associate Professor and Leader, Section of Cancer Biology, Hormel Institute, University of Minnesota.
- Interactions of Echinacea with Chemotherapy, Dr. Fathi Halaweish Associate Professor of Chemistry, South Dakota State University.
- "Yoga, Meditation, and the Ideals of Preventive Medicine." Dr. Rolf Sovik, clinical psychologist and co-director of the Himalayan Institute of Buffalo, New York.

In addition, in 2006, the Complementary and Integrative Medicine Program began sponsoring live telecasts of the *Integrative Medicine Program Lecture Series* presented by *University of Texas MD Anderson Cancer Center.*

Topics covered here have included the following:

- "Nutraceutical Science versus Nutraceutical Nonsense: A Pharmacologist's Perspective." Robert A. Newman, PhD, Professor of Cancer Medicine (Pharmacology), Co-Director, Pharmaceutical Development Center, University of Texas M. D. Anderson Cancer Center, Houston, TX.
- "Why are Omega-3 Fatty Acids Chemoprotective?" Robert S. Chapkin, PhD, Professor, University Faculty Fellow, & Director, Genomics & Bioinformatics Facility Core, Center for Environmental & Rural Health, Texas A&M University, College Station, TX.
- "Effects of acupuncture on human cerebro-cerebellar activity by fMRI", Kathleen Hui, MD, Assistant Neuroscientist, MGH NMR Center, Department of Radiology, Massachusetts General Hospital, Boston, MA.

An especially noteworthy achievement in 2004 was the creation of a curriculum in Integrative Medicine for the Mayo Graduate School Internal Medicine Residency. This curriculum was created to provide a broad overview of Integrative Medicine to resident physicians in training and will be delivered via a unique electronic format that permits asynchronous learning in a variety of settings.

9.2.2 Patient Care

An integrative medicine consult service was established in 2004. Dr. Ann Vincent, a Mayo-trained internist with advanced training in Women's Health, leads this service. In addition, Dr. Vincent has completed the Integrative Medicine Fellowship from the University of Arizona under Dr. Andrew Weil's leadership. Dr. Vincent is using this unique blend of skills to provide consults to patients at Mayo who have an interest in, or who are already using, Integrative Medicine modalities. Thus, physicians who are faced with a patient using a variety of herbs, for example, can refer that patient to Dr. Vincent for a thorough review of the herbs, identification of any potential drug/herb interactions and receive final recommendations regarding safe usage.

Data from 2005 show that over 300 patients were seen with 78% being female and the median age being 56 years with a range of 22–83 years. The most common reasons for patient referral are the following:

- Dietary/herbal supplements.
- Cancer (therapies before or after treatments).
- Postoperative pain/nausea.
- Osteoarthritis.
- Back pain.
- Headaches/migraines.
- Obesity.
- Fibromyalgia.
- Stress management.

Direct, frequent communications were critical to establishing the Consult Service. Leaders from the Program presented at Division and Department practice meetings throughout the institution. The Complementary and Integrative Medicine Program website was enhanced to convey specific and relevant information about the service as well as how to schedule appointments. A special ordering button was created on the Electronic Orders system used by all providers at Mayo Clinic. This allows request of a consult with a mouse click. In addition, ongoing presentations to staff and patient groups have helped maintain visibility of the service. The educational events also continue to provide both visibility and information about complementary medicine to a wide variety of staff.

Most recently, in 2006, approval from the Clinical Practice Committee was received to create a position for a licensed massage therapist. The massage therapist has initially been focusing on postoperative patients, with outcome measures suggestive of reduced pain and anxiety. Further expansion to other services is planned as resources permit. Acupuncture has been available at Mayo since the 1970s and has been delivered by physicians certified/licensed in acupuncture. Along with the massage therapist position, permission was also received to create a position for a licensed acupuncturist as well. As with the other clinical services, specific outcome measures will be collected to assess the results of these new services, to allow informed decisions regarding expansion of such services to other patient care areas.

9.3 Conclusion

Mayo Clinic has a long-standing reputation for commitment to evidenced-based practice and excellent patient care. Accordingly, the Cancer Center, faced with an increasing number of patients either using or interested in using a variety of therapies that had not been fully evaluated, responded with a focused program of research, the goal of which has been to place evidence-based information in the hands of clinicians and patients. The number of publications attests to the success of that goal. At the same time, members of the Cancer Center remain committed to the primary value that the needs of the patient come first. To this end, clinical interventions (e.g., consults and stress management education) and educational venues and programs have been incorporated in collaboration with colleagues from other disciplines at Mayo Clinic. As evidence accumulates, other services will be incorporated that can help meet the needs of our patients. Challenges of reimbursement and access remain which will hopefully be addressed as scientific evidence further delineates the proper role of these various interventions.

References

1. Harris PF, Remington PL, Trentham-Dietz A, Allen CI, Newcomb PA. Prevalence and treatment of menopausal symptoms among breast cancer survivors. J Pain Symptom Manage, 2002; 6:501–509.
2. Barton DL, Loprinzi CL, Quella SK, Sloan JA, Veeder MH, Egner JR, et al. Prospective evaluation of vitamin E for hot flashes in breast cancer survivors. J Clin Oncol 1998;16:495–500.
3. Quella SK, Loprinzi CL, Barton DL, Knost JA, Sloan JA, LaVasseur BI, et al. Evaluation of soy phytoestrogens for the treatment of hot flashes in breast cancer survivors: A North Central Cancer Treatment Group Trial. J Clin Oncol 2000;18:1068–1074.
4. Pockaj BA, Loprinzi CL, Sloan JA, Novotny PJ, Barton DL, Hagenmaier A, et al. Pilot evaluation of black cohosh for the treatment of hot flashes in women. Cancer Invest 2004;22:515–521.
5. Pockaj BA, Gallagher, J., Loprinzi, CL, Stella PJ, Barton DL, et al. Phase III double blinded randomized trial to evaluate the use of black cohosh in the treatment of hot flashes: A NCCTG study. J Clin Oncol, 2006;24:2836–2841.
6. Sloan JA, Loprinzi CL, Novotny PJ, Barton DL, Lavassseur BI, Windschitl H. Methodological lessons learned from hot flash studies. J Clin Oncol 2001;19:4280–4429
7. Barton DL, Loprinzi C, Atherton P, Carpenter L, Collins M, Carpenter P, et al. Dehydroepiandrosterone (DHEA) for the treatment of hot flashes: A pilot study. Support Cancer Ther 2006;3:91–97.
8. Vincent A., Barton DL, Mandrekar JN, et al. Acupuncture for hot flashes: A randomized sham-controlled clinical study. Menopause, 2007;14(1)45–52.
9. Ellison N, Loprinzi CL, Kugler J, Hatfield AK, Miser A, Sloan JA, et al. Phase III placebo-controlled trial of capsaicin cream in the management of surgical neuropathic pain in cancer patients. J Clin Oncol 1997;15:2974–2980.
10. Loprinzi CL, Kuross SA, O'Fallon JR, Gesme DH, Gerstner JB, Rospond RM, et al. Randomized placebo-controlled evaluation of hydrazine sulfate in patients with advanced colorectal cancer. J Clin Oncol 1994;12:1121–1125.

11. Loprinzi CL, Goldberg RM, Su JQ, Mailliard JA, Kuross SA, Maksymiuk AW, et al. Placebo-controlled trial of hydrazine sulfate in patients with newly diagnosed non-small cell lung cancer. J Clin Oncol 1997;12:1126–1129.
12. Jatoi A, Rowland K, Loprinzi CL, Sloan JA, Dakhil, SR, MacDonald N, et al. An eicosapentaenoic acid supplement versus megestrol acetate versus both for patients with cancer-associated wasting: A North Central Cancer Treatment Group and National Cancer Institute for Canada Collaborative Effort. J Clin Oncol 2004;22:2469–2476.
13. Moertel CG, Fleming TR, Kvols RJ, Sarna G, Koch R, Currie VE, et al. A clinical trial of amygdalin (Laetrile) in the treatment of human cancer. N Engl J Med 1982;306:201–206.
14. Creagan ET, Moertel CG, O'Fallon JR, Schutt AJ, O'Connell MJ, Rubin J, et al. Failure of high-dose vitamin C (ascorbic acid) therapy to benefit patients with advanced cancer. N Engl J Med 1979;301:687–690.
15. Jatoi A, Ellison N, Burch PA, Sloan JA, Dakhil SR, Novotny P, et al. A phase II trial of green tea in the treatment of patients with androgen independent metastatic prostate carcinoma. Cancer 2003;97:1442–1446.
16. Lane W, Comac L. Sharks don't get cancer: How sharks cartilage could save your life. Avery Publishing Group; 1992.
17. Loprinzi CL, Levitt R, Barton DL, Sloan JA, Atherton PJ, Smith DJ, et al. Evaluation of shark cartilage in patients with advanced cancer: A North Central Cancer Treatment Group Trial. Cancer 2005;104:176–182.
18. Mahood DJ, Dose AM, Loprinzi CL Veeder MH, Athmann LM, Therneau TM, et al. Inhibition of Fluorouracil-induced stomatitis by oral cryotherapy. J Clin Oncol 1991;9:449–452.
19. Rocke LK, Loprinzi CL, Lee JK, Kunselman SJ, Iverson RK, Finck G, et al A randomized clinical trial of two different durations of oral cryotherapy for prevention of 5-fluorouracil-related stomatitis. Cancer 1993;72:2234–2238.
20. Fidler P, Loprinzi CL, O'Fallon JR, Leitch JM, Lee JK, Hayes DL, et al. Prospective evaluation of a chamomile mouthwash for prevention of 5-FU-induced oral mucositis. Cancer 1996;77:522–525.
21. Loprinzi CL, Wender DB, Veeder MH, O'Fallon JR, Vaught NL, Dose AM, et al. Inhibition of 5-Fluorouracil-induced ocular irritation by ocular ice packs. Cancer 1994;74:945–948.
22. Okuno SH, Foote RL, Olmscheid MA, Sloan J, Sapiente RA, Novotny PJ, et al. Evaluation of an oral capsaicin lozenge for preventing radiation-induced mucositis. Journal of Cancer Integrative Medicine 2004;2:179–183.
23. Williams MS, Burk M, Loprinzi CL, Hill M, Schomberg JP, Nearhood K, et al. Phase III double-blind evaluation of an aloe vera gel as a prophylactic agent for radiation-induced skin toxicity. Int J Radiat Oncol Biol Phys 1996;36:345–349.
24. Loprinzi CL, Kugler JW, Sloan JA, Rooke TW, Quella SK, Novotny PJ, et al. Lack of effect of coumarin in women with lymphedema after treatment for breast cancer. New Engl J Med 1999;340:346–350.

The Research

Chapter 10
Mind–Body Research in Cancer

Kavita D. Chandwani, Alejandro Chaoul-Reich, Kelly A. Biegler, and Lorenzo Cohen

Contents

10.1 Utilization of Mind-Body Practices 140
10.2 Mind-Body Connection 141
10.3 Mind-Body Research at M. D. Anderson 143
10.4 Limitations of Mind-Body Research.. 153
References 154

Abstract Mind-body practices are defined as a variety of techniques designed to enhance the mind's capacity to affect bodily function and symptoms. A large percentage of the population, and especially people with cancer, participate in mind-body programs to help relieve stress, improve quality of life, and modulate physiological systems. At The University of Texas M. D. Anderson Cancer Center, we are conducting a number of clinical trials examining the biobehavioral effects of mind-body programs such as Tibetan Yoga, Hatha Yoga, meditation, and Qigong. Initial studies have found that these programs help to improve aspects of patient quality of life during and after treatment. More research is needed in this area with the use of appropriate control groups and thorough examination of the potential mediators of the benefits of the interventions to truly know the efficacy of these programs. It is clear that different mind-body practices have their place in oncology care. However, it is still uncertain which programs are most effective, and it will likely turn out that different programs are useful for different people at different times within the treatment and recovery trajectory. The key for health care professionals and patients is to encourage participation in some type of mind-body program to help improve aspects of quality of life.

Keywords: Mind-body medicine · oncology · quality of life · Yoga · meditation · Qigong.

L. Cohen
Director, Integrative Medicine Program, M. D. Anderson Cancer Center, 1515 Holcombe Blvd., Unit # 145, Houston, TX 77030
e-mail: lcohen@mdanderson.org

Mind-body practices are defined as a variety of techniques designed to enhance the mind's capacity to affect bodily function and symptoms [1]. Mind-body techniques include relaxation, hypnosis, visual imagery, meditation, biofeedback, cognitive-behavioral therapies, group support, autogenic training, and spirituality and expressive arts therapies such as art, music, or dance. Therapies such as Yoga, Tai chi, and Qigong often fall into the complementary and alternative medicine (CAM) category of energy medicine, as they are intended to work with bodily "energetic fields" (e.g., meridians and *qi* (pronounced chee—China), *lung* (pronounced loong—Tibet), *prana* (India), and *ki* (pronounced kee—Japan). However, they are likely to exert strong effects through a mind-body connection and as such fall into the mind-body medicine category. Some of these therapies are no longer considered "alternative" and they are well integrated into conventional medicine and most medical settings (hypnosis, biofeedback, cognitive-behavioral therapy, and group support). As research continues, the treatments that are found beneficial will hopefully become integrated into conventional medical care.

Mind-body techniques have been practiced in different parts of the world for thousands of years. This is especially true in the Eastern hemisphere, where the importance of the mind in illness and healing has been integral for more than 2000 years. This chapter briefly reviews the background on aspects of mind-body medicine and then focuses on the ongoing mind-body research we are conducting at The University of Texas M. D. Anderson Cancer Center (M. D. Anderson).

10.1 Utilization of Mind-Body Practices

Interest in mind-body medicine has been growing worldwide, parallel to the interest in other areas of CAM [2]. A nationwide survey found that 30% of the adult U.S. population indicated ever having used a mind-body technique, and 19% had used a mind-body technique within the past year [3]. In a recent survey among adults with and without cancer, use of mind-body techniques was reported to be about 26% [4]. Surveys of our patients at M. D. Anderson indicated that over 48% of patients had used mind-body techniques and 80% said they combined them with their cancer treatment [5].

Increasing awareness of the benefits of mind-body techniques to reduce stress has been fueled by celebrity participation and media-driven exposure to mind-body science with recent articles in The Wall Street Journal (January 19, 2007) and Time Magazine (January 29, 2007), and regular coverage on the topic by Newsweek (December 2002; November 2003; September 2004), Time Magazine (April 2001; January 2003; August 2003), National Geographic (March 2005), and most national newspapers (New York Times, Wall Street Journal, Washington Post, etc.). Most fitness centers around the nation offer some form of mind-body technique usually in the form of Yoga or Tai chi. Many corporate businesses and other employers offer relaxation, Yoga, or meditation classes and/or workshops to their staff. In the past decade, there has been a proliferation of Yoga studios, other forms of mind-body therapies, and wellness centers around the nation indicating the increased interest in the general population.

Mind-body practices such as meditation and Yoga have become extremely popular as a way to reduce stress and enhance spiritual growth. This is especially true for medical populations. Many cancer patients believe that stress plays a role in the etiology and progression of their disease. Some studies suggest that stressful life events may contribute to the incidence and progression of cancer [6], however, others have not found this association [7]. Although this research is equivocal, depression, which is a common psychological response to stressful life events or circumstances, has been linked to an increased risk of cancer and progression of disease [8, 9]. In support of this association, extensive research has now established that stress and depression cause suppression of cell-mediated immunity [10, 11] and are associated with increased angiogenesis in human and animal studies [12, 13], both of which are important factors involved with metastasis. A particularly important finding in this regard comes from prospective and cross-sectional studies in patients with breast cancer revealing that distress was negatively correlated with immune cell numbers and function after controlling for factors such as stage of disease and age [14, 15]. In addition, an association between survival time of breast cancer patients and both sympathetic nervous system activity and the patients' self-reported mental health has been reported [9, 16]. The biological and clinical significance of the influence of psychosocial factors on biological mechanisms and disease outcomes is only just starting to be understood. However, patients are already integrating mind-body techniques within their conventional medical care to help manage stress.

10.2 Mind-Body Connection

The belief that what we think and feel can influence our health and has a place in healing dates back thousands of years [17]. The importance of the role of the mind, emotions, and behaviors in health and well-being was part of traditional Chinese, Tibetan, and Ayurvedic medicine and other medical traditions of the world. Hippocrates is said to have received his medical training at an Asclepieion temple (healing temple), where the followers of Asclepius, the Greek god of medicine and healing, believed in the moral and spiritual aspects of healing and that treatment could occur only with consideration of attitude, environmental influences, and natural remedies (approximately 400 B.C.). The integrated approach to health and medicine was maintained in Eastern medical systems, but during the Renaissance and Enlightenment eras in the West, there was a separation between mind and body in relation to the role of the mind in medicine. With the advent of many scientific discoveries and technological advances (e.g., bacteria, antibiotics, and advanced surgical techniques), the role of the mind in medicine went by the wayside and modern Western medicine simply focused on the body to the exclusion of the mind. This long-held belief is slowly dissipating as there is mounting scientific evidence demonstrating that what we think and feel can definitely influence our physiology, biology, and health. There is now also ample evidence to show that our biological systems also influence how we think, feel, and behave.

The work of Cannon [18] and Seyle [19] early in the 20th century demonstrated that psychological stress can have a profound influence on physiological systems, thus demonstrating a possible role for stress and disease, and, therefore, health and well-being. The early work of Pavlov [20] also demonstrated that psychological processes taking place in the brain, namely conditioning, can also influence biological processes in the body. The subsequent work by Ader and Cohen [21] showed that the immune system could also be conditioned to a previously neutral stimulus, demonstrating that the immune system, and for that matter most biological systems, can be influenced by psychological processes. We now know that psychological processes can influence physiological systems, and these changes can in turn affect disease states [22].

In the West, pioneering research in mind-body medicine conducted by Benson and Kabat-Zinn [23,24] helped to form the scientific field. Early research by Benson et al. [23,25] found that the practice of Transcendental Meditation (TM) resulted in lowered blood pressure, reduction in oxygen consumption, heart rate, and metabolic rate, greater than is expected during sleep, with an increase in alpha waves. All these changes indicated a state of relaxation where there was diminished sympathetic nervous system activity following meditation. Benson coined the term the "relaxation response."

Benson and colleagues [26] subsequently investigated three advanced practitioners of the Tibetan meditative practice called *tum-mo*, who were living in the lower Himalayas. Practitioners of *tum-mo* claim to increase their body temperature through a special meditative technique of deep concentration. Traditionally, these practices are done in a very cold environment with minimal clothes on the practitioners' body to see if they could dry a wet sheet at under 40°F and then wet the dry sheet by the perspiration of their body as they continued performing the *tum-mo* practice. In the cold environment, the advanced *tum-mo* practitioners could increase the temperature of their fingers and toes by as much as 8.3°C [26]. A significant reduction in their oxygen consumption was also observed.

Kabat-Zinn developed a combination of *Vipassana* (a Buddhist mindfulness meditation technique), some Yoga postures, and a body scan technique in a behavioral medicine setting for populations with various types of chronic pain [27, 28]. Originally called Stress Reduction and Relaxation Program (SR-RP), and later coined as Mindfulness-Based Stress Reduction (MBSR), it was described as "paying attention in a particular way: on purpose, in the present moment, and nonjudgementally" [29]. MBSR has been extensively scientifically investigated in the West and is useful for helping to ease psychological and physical effects of some chronic illnesses [30, 31].

Research has shown that after being diagnosed with cancer, patients try to bring about positive changes in their lifestyles, indicating a tendency to take control of their health care [32]. Techniques of stress management that have proven helpful include progressive muscle relaxation [33, 34], diaphragmatic breathing

[35, 36], guided imagery [37–39], social support [40, 41], and meditation [42, 43]. Participating in stress management programs prior to treatment have enabled patients to tolerate therapy with fewer reported side effects [44–47]. Supportive expressive group therapy has also been found to be useful for patients with cancer [48–50]. Psychosocial interventions have been shown to specifically decrease depression and anxiety and to increase self-esteem and active-approach coping strategies [51–53].

10.3 Mind-Body Research at M. D. Anderson

At M. D. Anderson, pilot studies of mind-body interventions have been conducted in various cancer populations including lymphoma and breast cancer during or after treatment. There are a number of ongoing studies funded by The National Institutes of Health, investigating the effects of Yoga (from the Indian and Tibetan traditions), meditation, and Qigong.

10.3.1 Background on Yoga, Meditation, and Qigong

10.3.1.1 Yoga

Yoga is an ancient mind-body science that has been practiced for millennia. The word "Yoga" comes from the Sanskrit meaning "to yoke" or join [54]. The form of Yoga we are most familiar with in the West comes from India. Many varieties of similar mind-body techniques also existed and were practiced in other areas of Asia such as Tibet, China, and Japan.

Patanjali formally described the practice of Yoga in the treatise *Yoga Sutras* over 2000 years ago [55]. He defined Yoga as the process of eliminating thoughts from the mind and allowing it to settle down to silence in a relaxed and clear state. Attaining such a balance helps a person develop a balanced and healthy mind and body. Yoga incorporates various postures/movements (*asana*), breathing techniques (such as *pranayama*), visual imagery, meditation, and relaxation techniques.

Similar techniques have been also practiced for thousands of years in other parts of Asia including *Tsa lung* and *Trul khor* in Tibet [what we call Tibetan yoga (TY) in the West] and Qigong in China. There are many similarities between these Eastern practices including specialized breathing techniques, mindfulness practices, and body movements all with a focus on training and harmonizing of one's "life force" or "vital breath" (*prana* (India), *lung* (Tibet), *or qi* (China). Tibetan *Tsa lung trul khor* is better translated from the Tibetan as "magical movements." It is a distinctive Tibetan practice of physical Yoga in which breath and concentration of the mind are integrated as crucial components in conjunction with particular body movements, and thus is known as Tibetan yoga. Contemporary Tibetan religious leaders and scholars describe magical movement practices as dating back to at least the 8th century [56].

There are many misconceptions about Yoga in the Western world as it is often considered a form of exercise or gymnastics (twisting the body into a pretzel) or even a religion. In the West more emphasis has been also placed on the *asana*, with less of a focus on *pranayama* and meditation. Due to the mental and physical aspects of Yoga, a quintessential mind-body program, it may be particularly useful for cancer patients early in the diagnosis and treatment process or moving into post-treatment period.

The physical and mental health benefits of Yoga have been described in early texts [54, 57–59]. Although it has been used in India to treat disease for centuries [60], this aspect has only recently started gaining recognition in the West. There has been an interest in the therapeutic applications of Yoga over the past 30 years [61–68]. However, Yoga was often incorporated as only one aspect of a multicomponent intervention program (e.g., Yoga, diet, and support groups) making it difficult to know the true contribution of Yoga itself. In chronically ill populations, Yoga has lessened the severity of musculoskeletal disease [58,69], decreased the frequency and duration of epileptic seizures [70], decreased the frequency and severity of asthma attacks [71], improved peak expiratory flow rate in bronchial asthmatics [72], improved the lipid profile of patients with coronary artery disease [73], and effectively controlled aspects of hypertension [74].

In healthy populations, Yoga-based interventions have been shown to decrease depression and anxiety [68, 75], increase motor control [76, 77], and improve subjective measures of well-being [78] and quality of life (QOL). A randomized controlled trial of a Yoga intervention among medical students found that students who participated in the Yoga-based intervention experienced decreased depression and anxiety and increased empathy and spirituality when compared with those in the control group [79]. There have also been a number of studies suggesting that Yoga produces acute physiological changes [80–84].

The first study of Yoga in a population of cancer patients recruited 125 patients undergoing radiotherapy to participate in group therapy, meditation, or Yoga [85]. They found Yoga to be useful in improving QOL during radiotherapy and for some time immediately after completion of radiotherapy. The patients reported increased appetite, increased tolerance to radiotherapy, improved sleep, improved bowel habits, and a feeling of peace and tranquility. Improved disease coping has been reported among inpatients suffering from various malignancies who participated in Yoga that was offered in conjunction with autogenous relaxation training, psychotherapeutic services, or both [86]. Although this program was not conducted within a research framework, they reported improvements in movement, lymphatic drainage, speech therapy, pain control, and overall psychosocial care in terms of achieving "inner calmness and relaxation."

10.3.1.2 Meditation

Meditation, which is often incorporated as a component of Yoga, has been defined in various ways and perhaps depends on the tradition and background of the practitioners. According to the ancient Hindu sage Patanjali, *dhyana* (meditation) involves training the mind to concentrate on an internal or external object and followed by concentration on the internal perception of the object until the mind gains control over "everything" [87].

From the Buddhist tradition, it is stated that Buddha Shakyamuni defined meditation (*bhavana*) as a state of "mental health" or "mental culture" that is in equilibrium and tranquility [88] (pp. 67–8). Through meditation one can cleanse the mind of impurities and disturbances and cultivate such qualities as concentration, awareness, intelligence, joy, tranquility, and wisdom [88]. There are two "classic" forms of meditation in the Buddhist tradition: (1) Quiescence (*shamata*), defined as meditative concentration (*samadhi*) that has the characteristic of mental single-pointedness and (2) Insight (*vipassana*), defined as wisdom (*prajna*) that has the nature of thorough knowledge of reality. Insight is an analytical meditative method based on mindfulness, awareness, vigilance, and observation [88, 89] (p. 69).

Meditation has been investigated in healthy and medical populations and is probably the most investigated mind-body practice. There are various types of meditations that are practiced in the West; some of them include TM, Vipassana meditation, Brahmakumari's meditation, Tibetan Meditation, Sudarshan Kriya, and Om-meditation.

Transcendental Meditation.

Initiated by Maharishi Mahesh Yogi, TM involves a word, phrase, or a mantra suitable to a person, repeated mentally while sitting in a comfortable position for 20 min. The meditator is instructed to prevent distracting thoughts. Early studies of TM have found it was associated with reduction of chronic pain, high blood pressure, serum cholesterol, substance abuse, and anxiety, and with improvements in QOL [90–98]. Although the specific mechanisms by which meditation relieves pain are not well understood, recent neuroimaging studies have observed a reduction of activity in certain brain regions relevant to pain sensation when externally applied painful stimulus was delivered to long-term practitioners and new learners of TM [99]. Some studies have also found elevated nighttime melatonin levels associated with meditation in healthy individuals [100].

Mindfulness-Based Stress Reduction

MBSR [24], developed by Jon Kabat-Zinn, has participants meet weekly for 2–2.5 h each time for 8–10 weeks complemented by an all day (7–8 h) intensive practice session, usually planned around the 6th week. Participants also have homework practice (45 min per day, 6 days per week) and behavioral assignments [24, 27, 28]. This structured program draws from several Eastern traditions and is a combination of theory as well as practice of mindfulness, similar to that taught by Buddhist and Zen monks, body scan, and hatha Yoga from the Indian tradition [27]. Mindfulness meditation has been shown to be an effective coping technique for patients with stress disorders, chronic pain, and various chronic diseases [30, 31, 101–103]. Although this well-structured program has been applied to many populations with the aim of coping with suffering that arises from clinical and non-clinical problems, it is not clear what the key components are as the multi-component program comes from many Eastern traditions.

Davidson et al. [104] also reported neurophysiological changes in novice meditators who were trained in MBSR. The meditation-trained group showed significant reductions in anxiety and negative affect immediately after completing the 8-week MBSR program. In addition, the meditation-trained group displayed significantly greater left lateralized anterior activation compared to controls 4 months after MBSR training, which is consistent with other findings indicating a positive relationship between positive affect and increased left anterior activity [104–107]. This study also demonstrated a clear association between the brain and the immune system, as the meditation-trained participants also exhibited a significantly larger antibody titer response to an influenza vaccine injection following meditation training, which was positively correlated with left anterior activity.

Lutz et al. [108] investigated neural synchrony in expert meditators and controls during both resting and meditative states. Neural synchrony, as indexed by EEG, has been shown to reflect the simultaneous function of several cortical structures during higher order cognition including attention and working memory [109–112]. Compared to controls, expert meditators showed greater neural synchrony over frontal-parietal regions during baseline states, which further increased during a meditative state over frontolateral and posterior regions. The amount of practice, rather than age, contributed to the neural synchrony differences observed between expert meditators and controls. However, the results suggest that neural synchrony can develop with meditation practice. The neural plasticity of the brain that is demonstrated in these studies opens up a whole area of research in relation to cognition, emotion, physiology, biology, behavior, and health.

A cognitive dimension was added to MBSR by Teasdale, Segal, and Williams [113] with the premise that the skills of attentional control taught in mindfulness meditation with cognitive therapy skills could be helpful in preventing relapse of major depressive episodes. This program has been called Mindfulness-Based Cognitive Therapy (MBCT). This modification in MBSR has been reported to be effective in reducing depression relapse [114].

A few studies have begun to examine MBSR in an oncology setting. Speca et al. [115] randomly assigned 109 patients with early- and late-stage cancer either to a 7-week intervention group that included group support and discussion, mindfulness meditation, visualization and imagery, and Yoga stretches or to a wait list control group. At the end of the 7-week program, participants in the intervention group experienced lower total mood disturbance and decreased overall distress compared to those in the control group. Carlson et al. [116] conducted a trial that examined the benefits of mindfulness meditation in an outpatient oncology population and found the program to be effective in decreasing mood disturbance and stress symptoms by the end of the intervention. More recently, Carlson and colleagues [117] have also reported significant improvements in sleep quality and reduction in mood disturbances and fatigue in a heterogeneous group of cancer patients practicing MBSR. A small non-randomized correlational study of women with breast cancer found higher overnight melatonin levels for those practicing MBSR (5–7 sessions per week for 30–45 min) compared to women with breast cancer not practicing MBSR [43].

10.3.1.3 Qigong

Qi is a term that has been used in Chinese for millennia to describe energy that runs throughout the human body and is equivalent to the concept of "life force" or *prana* in India and *lung* in Tibet. Qi runs along meridians or channels that run through different parts of the body. As qi is considered to be similar to energy, it can be dynamic, stagnant, blocked, created, and even radiated. Within the body it is thought that good health is the result of unblocked qi that naturally runs throughout the body. Blockages of qi can cause varied symptoms ranging from mood disturbances to physical morbidities. By relieving this blockage and allowing qi to flow naturally, the problem will be remedied and the body will return to a balanced state [118–120].

Qigong is composed of two terms: "*qi*" energy flow and "*gong*" meaning skill or achievement [121]. The four main components of Qigong include training in consciousness, breathing, body movement, and adjustment or stimulation of one's own qi. The various forms Qigong has taken depend on the intended use of manipulating qi. These different forms include scholar, martial, medical, and spiritual.

The Tientsin Chinese Medicine Academy has suggested applying different styles of Qigong for different medical conditions [118]. Qigong for general health maintenance may be practiced for as little as 20 min a day, 3–4 h for mild diseases, and 8–12 h for serious diseases. A typical daily Qigong session consists of five elements: meditation, cleansing qi, strengthening qi, circulating qi, and dispersing qi [121].

Qigong practice consists primarily of meditation, relaxation, guided imagery, and building energy through mind-body integration of specific postures, breathing techniques, and a mindful focus on areas of the body. The practice of Qigong as a therapeutic means of achieving and maintaining health are based on the holistic concept that nature and man form an organic whole.

Studies of Qigong have included psychosocial, physical, and physiological outcomes. These studies have employed a variety of types of Qigong including Tai chi chuan (see below). Some studies included control groups and others were case reports or single-arm trials. Most studies to date have been published in the Chinese literature, and few studies have examined the benefits of Qigong for patients with cancer. In clinical trials, Qigong has been reported to significantly reduce the side effects of medical therapies [122, 123], anxiety [123–126], and pain [123] and significantly increase self-efficacy [127] and sleep quality [128, 129].

Physiologically, Qigong has been found to lower blood pressure, norepinephrine, epinephrine, and cortisol levels [129, 130]. Other studies have reported a 50% increase in the CD4/CD8 T lymphocyte ratio in a Qigong trainee group compared to those who did not practice [131], increased adhesion capacity of neutrophils, increased neutrophil function through examination of superoxide generation, and increased NK cell cytotoxicity [126, 132]. A pilot study of Qigong of Guolin lineage in healthy subjects found decreased cortisol levels and increased interferon (IFN)

γ-secreting cells and decreased interleukin (IL)10-secreting cells in Phytohemagglutin PHA-stimulated cultures, increasing the IFNγ:IL10 ratio [133]. Changes in cholesterol levels and changes in the metabolism of lipids have been observed in some studies comparing a Qigong intervention to a control group [129, 134].

Tai chi, a form of martial Qigong, is practiced on the premise that qi is generated in the body and guided to the limbs to increase power. This practice involves minimal muscle usage and a soft technique. Tai chi has been found to improve sleep quality [128], improve physical functioning [135], and increase immunity to varicella-zoster virus [136]. Lung function has also improved, with increases in ventilatory efficiency for oxygen uptake and carbon dioxide production, as well as general breathing patterns [137, 138]. Similarly, Tai chi delayed the decline of cardiorespiratory function of older individuals [139].

Only one study has been conducted in the United States for patients with cancer, and they investigated the influence of Tai chi in breast cancer survivors. Twenty-one breast cancer survivors were randomized to receive 12 weeks of Tai chi or psychosocial support therapy (PST), three times a week. Participants in the Tai chi group reported increased functional capacity such as increased aerobic capacity, muscular strength, and flexibility while those in the PST group reported only increased flexibility [140]. The investigators also found that the women in the Tai chi group reported increased health-related QOL as well as increased self esteem, while those in the PST group reported declines in both areas [141]. These reports suggest that participation in this form of Qigong is beneficial to breast cancer survivors in the areas of functional capacity and health-related QOL.

10.3.2 M. D. Anderson's Past and Ongoing Studies of Yoga, Meditation, and Qigong

10.3.2.1 Yoga

Two initial studies conducted by our group examined the effects of Tibetan Yoga. For these pilot studies, a seven-session program called "Tibetan Yoga" (TY) was designed and included practices from the Tibetan Bon tradition, included in the Mother Tantra *(Ma rgyud)* and Great Completeness Oral Transmission of Zhang Zhung (*Zhang zhung snyan rgyud*). The intervention, chosen in consultation with Tenzin Wangyal Rinpoche of the Ligmincha Institute, consisted of four main components: (1) breathing exercises, (2) meditative concentration, (3) *tsa-lung* sitting yogic postures, and (4) *trul-khor* yogic postures involving more physical movement. These components have been used in the Bon tradition for centuries and we chose them with the intention that they would help in ameliorating side effects and hastening recovery for patients who were either undergoing active treatment or who had recently completed treatment.

The breathing exercises help participants to regulate their breath and prepare for the movement-based practice. The breathing techniques are thought to help calm the mind and manage physical, emotional, and mental "obstacles." The meditative concentration techniques the patients learned helped them to use the calmness of the mind toward self-observation and to guide the breath to clear away obstacles. They also learned a simple meditative technique that incorporated sound and visualization. The *tsa lung* exercises applied the meditative concentration techniques, and the breathing exercises already learned with five specific simple movements focused in different areas of the body at points called *chakras* (located at the head, neck, chest, lower abdomen, and perineum), to help participants relax and feel invigorated. The first five movements from the *trul khor* were then introduced and again the participants used the meditative concentration techniques and the breathing exercises while performing the simple movements. All the techniques were done either sitting on a cushion on the floor or sitting in a chair. The classes were taught by an instructor authorized by the Ligmincha Institute. The hour-long classes were taught once a week for 7 weeks. This provided the participants the opportunity to learn the techniques and practice them with the instructor, so that they could continue to practice them on their own. At the end of each class, the participants received printed material to take home and use as support of the techniques learned in that session. At the end of the course, the participants were given an audio tape with guided practices of all the techniques they learnt. Participants were advised to continue daily practice at home in addition to the class at the clinic and also to continue their practice after the 7-week course was over. Patients completed measures of intrusive thoughts and avoidance behaviors (Impact of Events Scale: IES), depressive symptoms (Center for Epidemiological Studies – Depression: CES-D), sleep disturbances (Pittsburgh Sleep Quality Index: PSQI), fatigue (Brief Fatigue Inventory: BFI), and QOL (SF-36) at baseline, 1 week, and 1 and 3 months after the last class.

In the first pilot study, we examined the feasibility, acceptability, and initial efficacy of the TY program described above for patients with lymphoma. Thirty-nine patients were randomly assigned to either the TY group or to a wait listed control group. The intervention group received the 7-week TY program, and the wait list control group could receive the instruction after the end of the study. Patients had to be currently undergoing treatment or had to have completed treatment within the past 12 months.

There was an even distribution of severity of disease between the two groups and among those who were undergoing active treatment. We began the 7-week sessions after each recruitment cycle, which allowed us to teach the classes to four to nine people in each session. Eighty-nine percent of TY participants completed at least two to three Yoga sessions; 58 percent completed at least five sessions. Overall, the results indicated that the TY program was feasible and well liked by the patients. The majority of participants indicated that the program was "a little" or "definitely" beneficial, with no one indicating "not beneficial," and they continued practicing at least once a week, with many continuing to practice twice a week or more [142]. The study results indicated that the TY group reported lower overall sleep disturbances (5.8 vs. 8.1; $P < 0.004$) during the follow-up period than did the control group. Participants practicing Yoga had better sleep quality ($P < 0.02$), had less difficulty falling asleep ($P < 0.01$), slept significantly longer, and used fewer sleep medications ($P < 0.02$) than did those in the control group [142]. Improving sleep quality in a cancer population may be particularly salient as sleep is crucial for recovery. Fatigue and sleep disturbances are common problems for patients with cancer.

A second study examined the benefits of the same 7-week TY program for women with breast cancer. Women with stage I–III breast cancer who were undergoing active treatment (radiotherapy or chemotherapy) or who underwent treatment less than 1 year prior to enrollment were recruited to participate in the study. Fifty-nine women were randomized to either the Yoga group or a wait list control group. Initial analyses have been conducted and presented at national meetings [143].

On average, the participants in the TY group said they found the program useful or very useful, and they practiced it around twice a week. A mixed model analysis, controlling for the dependent variable at baseline, revealed a group by time effect with respect to IES total scores ($P = 0.03$). Descriptive statistics and a graphical display of the data indicated that the Yoga group reported lower IES scores than the control group by the 3-month assessment (adjusted means: 17.1 vs. 20.1). A multivariate linear regression, controlling for baseline, revealed that the Yoga group reported lower scores for cancer-related symptoms at the 1-week follow-up than the control group (change in means: –8.1 vs. 3.9, $P = 0.04$). This study was underpowered for extensive analyses; however, again the means were in the expected direction. The results of this second study indicated that the TY program was feasible and well-liked by women with breast cancer.

These pilot programs are among the few studies of Yoga in a cancer patient population and the only scientific studies of TY in any population. We are now conducting an NCI-funded trial (R01) examining the effects of TY for women with breast cancer undergoing chemotherapy. Women in the TY group are being compared to women who learn some simple stretching exercises and to women in a wait list control group.

A subsequent small randomized pilot trial examined the effects of Yoga from the Indian tradition for women with breast cancer undergoing radiation treatment at M. D. Anderson. Sixty-one women were either assigned to the Yoga group or a wait list control group that could participate in the Yoga after the study was completed. Patients in the Yoga group participated in the Yoga sessions twice a week for the duration of their radiotherapy, each session lasting about 1 hour. The Yoga program consisted of four main components: (1) various loosening exercises; (2) seven simple postures and a deep relaxation technique; (3) alternate nostril breathing; and (4) meditation. These techniques were developed by and chosen in consultation with the Swami Vivekananda Yoga Research Foundation, a Yoga research institution in Bangalore, India, with extensive clinical and research experience conducting this form of Yoga with healthy and medical populations [60, 72, 144]. The components were specifically designed and selected for use in patients with cancer, with particular emphasis on the problems that women experience while undergoing radiotherapy for breast cancer and recovering from surgery and/or chemotherapy. The overall aim of these techniques was to train the participants to regulate their breathing, be aware of the various changes that occur in the body while performing the maneuvers, and by doing so the participants can calm the mind and relax parts of the body. In the beginning, patients were introduced to each of the four different areas over a period of four 1-h classes conducted by a Vivekananda Yoga Research Foundation certified Instructor. During the remainder of the sessions, the participants practiced the complete program. The exercises were done to meet each patient's needs. At the end of each of the first four classes, the participants were given a CD with a recording of the technique they just learned and some printed materials that they could take home. After the fourth session, they were given a CD with all instructions as well as a complete printed version. Participants were advised to continue daily practice at home in addition to the class at the hospital and also after the completion of radiotherapy.

The loosening and breathing exercises consisted of various gentle, sometimes repetitive, movements of the arms, legs, neck, and eyes in standing, sitting, and supine positions. Postures, or *asanas*, were done standing, sitting, or lying down (either face down or face up). These postures consisted of simple movements that included a side bending posture, two forward bending postures, three back bending postures, and a partial shoulder stand with wall support. The session always ended with the supine relaxation posture to allow the body to relax completely. In this position, they practiced the deep relaxation technique that incorporated gentle sounds that would resonate their body (e.g. "aah," "uuu," "mmm," and "om"). Alternate nostril breathing was done for five rounds, sitting with the back and neck straight. Meditation was done sitting in any comfortable position or sitting on a chair. The patients were instructed to close their eyes and concentrate on their breath and their thoughts. They were then encouraged to repeat the syllable "mmm" mentally. They were instructed to sit in silence and dwell on a single positive thought of their choice. This could be continued for about 10-20 min.

Patients completed the IES, CES-D, PSQI, BFI, and SF-36 at baseline, 1 week, and 1 and 3 months after the last radiation therapy. Initial analyses have been conducted and presented at national meetings examining the 1-week post-radiation treatment, 1 week after the 6 weeks of Yoga classes. The results indicated that 1 week after the end of radiation treatment, the Yoga participants reported better physical functioning, (adjusted means: Yoga 81.8 vs. control 68.6, $P < 0.01$), significantly higher SF-36 general health scores (adjusted means: Yoga 78.3 vs. control 67.9, $P < 0.03$), marginally better SF-36 social functioning scores (adjusted means: Yoga 85.3 vs. control 76.0, $P > 0.1$), significantly lower levels of sleep-related daytime dysfunction (adjusted means: Yoga 0.5 vs. control 1.2, $P < 0.04$), and marginally lower levels of fatigue (adjusted means: Yoga 1.9 vs. control 3.1, $P < 0.06$) than the control group [145]. There were no other group differences on the SF-36 subscales or for the CES-D or IES scores. A similar study funded by the NCI (R21) is ongoing where the participants are randomized to one of three groups—Yoga group, stretching group, or a wait list control group. The follow-up study is examining the biobehavioral effects of the Yoga program using a more appropriate control group in order to separate the effects of Yoga from social support and simple stretching exercises.

10.3.2.2 Meditation

A mindfulness relaxation (MR) study headed by Dr. Jon Hunter from Mount Sinai Hospital, Toronto, Canada, is being conducted within the M. D. Anderson Community Clinical Oncology Program (CCOP). The purpose of the study is to test this behavioral intervention in reducing psychological and physiological side effects of chemotherapy in cancer patients. In this randomized trial, patients with newly diagnosed cancer, who are about to undergo chemotherapy, are randomly assigned to one of three groups: the MR group, a relaxing music (RM) group where participants listen to music for the same amount of time as the MR participants, or a standard care control group where participants receive standard medical education on chemotherapy (SC). Patients complete assessments before being randomized (baseline), in the middle of their course of chemotherapy, at the end of treatment, and 3 months after the end of treatment. They also complete very brief diary assessments for 3 days before the start of each cycle of chemotherapy and for 3 days after. Blood samples for immune indices are also being obtained.

The MR intervention consists of a script containing elements of relaxation induction, Yoga breathing, guided imagery, and a "mindful" attitude, which encourages people to become aware and take notice of physical sensations without having to alter or respond to them [28]. Nurses at each site are trained in the administration of the script, and subsequently deliver it to patients before their first chemotherapy session, in order to establish a pre-emptive association between relaxation and the chemotherapy setting, that will in turn diminish the development of conditioned symptoms. The patients are also given a CD of the MR recorded by the site nurse who delivered the MR training to use at home for practice sessions and for all chemotherapy sessions.

Each time the patient attends a chemotherapy session, the MR exercise is conducted prior to and during chemotherapy delivery, via use of a portable CD player with the recorded version. Participants are instructed to use the CD at home at least once daily throughout chemotherapy delivery in order to become familiar with and build skill in the technique. The participants in the RM group use a CD with RM. Patients in the RM group utilize their CD in a manner identical to the MR CD, but they do not receive any specific instructions on relaxation or meditation. They also receive general information on the management of symptoms related to chemotherapy in a session of equivalent time to the MR training session. The SC arm receives general information on the management of symptoms related to chemotherapy in the manner that is typical of that CCOP site. The single arm feasibility pilot trial went well and the large phase III randomized trial is now underway.

10.3.2.3 Qigong

An ongoing pilot project of Qigong is examining the initial efficacy of implementing a Qigong program for patients with breast cancer undergoing radiotherapy. This study is being conducted at the Fudan University Cancer Hospital, Shanghai, China as part of an International Center of Traditional Chinese Medicine for

Cancer funded by the NCI (U19). Patients with breast cancer who are undergoing radiotherapy are randomly assigned to either a Qigong group or a wait list control group. Participants in the Qigong group attend daily Qigong sessions 5 days/week throughout their 6-week radiotherapy schedule. The sessions are coordinated with the treatment schedule and conducted near the treatment facility. The patients are taught a modified version *Gualin Qigong* including preparation exercises [standing posture, breathing exercise, and opening and closing of the *dantian* (an important focus point for internal meditative techniques, located in the abdomen three finger widths below and two finger widths behind the navel)], main exercise (slow exercise and fast exercise), and then the closing exercise. The focus is on working with gentle movements and breath to help regulate the patients' *qi*. Measures are obtained prior to randomization, mid-way through radiotherapy, during last week of radiotherapy, and 1 and 3 months after the end of radiotherapy. To date, we have recruited and randomized 80 women. The recruiting procedures have gone well, patients are enthusiastic about participating in the research, and compliance with attending the Qigong sessions is excellent (>90%). Once we determine the initial efficacy of the Qigong program, we will conduct a larger randomized trial to validate the benefits of Qigong as an adjuvant to radiotherapy in patients with breast cancer in which we will include the appropriate control groups to examine components of the Qigong program and some of the possible mechanisms of action that could be indirect (e.g., attention and social support) and/or direct (e.g., relaxation and aspects of physical activity). A larger trial can also track the patients for a longer period of time.

10.4 Limitations of Mind-Body Research

Much of the current research in mind-body medicine and cancer is trying to determine the benefits of different types of interventions on physical, biological, and psychological outcomes. Ongoing research in this area making use of neuroimaging techniques [99, 108] and examining different biological processes [146, 147] clearly points to the major role that the mind can have in influencing health and well-being.

One of the limitations of mind-body research to date is that either no control groups were used or the control groups only received standard supportive care. The control groups did not receive any specific instruction from the medical staff, they did not meet in groups, and they did not receive any extra attention from the medical staff. We, therefore, do not know if the positive benefits from the intervention are unique to the intervention, for example, Yoga, or whether the same benefits could come from learning some simple stretching exercises, doing light physical activity or simple relaxation exercises, meeting in small groups, or simply getting extra attention from the medical staff. Ongoing research at M. D. Anderson and other institutions around the world will help to answer these questions through the inclusion of appropriate control groups. Moreover, there are many obstacles that are inherent in the measures being used, be it psychosocial self-report instruments or even problems such as noise interference in highly sophisticated equipment such as functional Magnetic Resonance Imaging.

Research of mind-body practices are starting to reveal the psychological, behavioral, physiological, and biological effects of these techniques. More clinical trials are clearly needed with appropriate control groups and thorough examination of the potential mediators of the benefits of the interventions to truly know the efficacy of these programs. It is clear that different mind-body practices have their place in oncology care. However, it is still uncertain which programs are most effective and it will likely turn out that different programs are useful for different people at different times within the treatment and recovery trajectory. The key for health care professionals and patients is to encourage participation in some type of mind-body program to help improve aspects of QOL.

References

1. NCCAM. Expanding Horizons of Health Care Strategic Plan 2005–2009: National Center for Complementary and Alternative Medicine; 2004.
2. Kessler RC, Davis RB, Foster DF, Van Rompay MI, Walters EE, Wilkey SA, et al. Long-term trends in the use of complementary and alternative medical therapies in the United States. Annals of Internal Medicine 2001 Aug 21;135(4):262–8.
3. Wolsko PM, Eisenberg DM, Davis RB, Phillips RS. Use of mind-body medical therapies. Journal of General Internal Medicine 2004;19(1):43–50.
4. Goldstein MS, Brown ER, Ballard-Barbash R, Morgenstern H, Bastani R, Lee J, et al. The use of complementary and alternative medicine among California adults with and without cancer. Evidence Based Complementary & Alternative Medicine: eCAM 2005;2(4): 557–65.
5. Richardson MA, Sanders T, Palmer JL, Greisinger A, Singletary SE. Complementary/alternative medicine use in a comprehensive cancer center and the implications for oncology. Journal of Clinical Oncology 2000;18(13):2505–14.
6. Chen CC, David AS, Nunnerley H, Michell M, Dawson JL, Berry H, et al. Adverse life events and breast cancer: Case-control study. British Medical Journal 1995;311:1527–30.
7. Petticrew M, Fraser JM, Regan MF. Adverse life-events and risk of breast cancer: A meta-analysis. British Journal of Health Psychology 1999;4:1–17.
8. Penninx BW, Guralnik JM, Pahor M, Ferrucci L, Cerhan JR, Wallace RB, et al. Chronically depressed mood and cancer risk in older persons. Journal of the National Cancer Institute 1998;90:1888–93.
9. Watson M, Haviland JS, Greer S, Davidson J, Bliss JM. Influence of psychological response on survival in breast cancer: A population-based cohort study. Lancet 1999;354(9187): 1331–6.
10. Irwin M, Patterson T, Smith TL, Caldwell C, Brown SA, Gillin JC, et al. Reduction of immune function in life stress and depression. Biological Psychiatry 1990;27:22–30.
11. Rabin BS. Stress, Immune Function, and Health: The Connection. New York, New York: Wiley-Liss & Sons; 1999.
12. Lutgendorf SK, Johnsen EL, Cooper B, Anderson B, Sorosky JI, Buller RE, et al. Vascular endothelial growth factor and social support in patients with ovarian carcinoma. Cancer 2002;95:808–15.
13. Thaker PH, Han LY, Kamat AA, Arevalo JM, Takahashi R, Lu C, et al. Chronic stress promotes tumor growth and angiogenesis in a mouse model of ovarian carcinoma. Nature Medicine 2006 Aug;12(8):939–44.

14. Andersen BL, Farrar WB, Golden-Kreutz D, Kutz LA, MacCallum R, Courtney ME, et al. Stress and immune responses after surgical treatment for regional breast cancer. Journal of the National Cancer Institute 1998;90(1):30–6.
15. Tjemsland L, Soreide JA, Matre R, Malt UF. Preoperative psychological variables predict immunological status in patients with operable breast cancer. Psycho-Oncology 1997;6: 311–20.
16. Sephton SE, Sapolsky RM, Kraemer HC, Spiegel D. Diurnal cortisol rhythm as a predictor of breast cancer survival. Journal of the National Cancer Institute 2000;92(12):994–1000.
17. Shankar K, Liao LP. Traditional systems of medicine. Physical Medicine and Rehabilitation Clinics of North America 2004;15(4):725–47.
18. Cannon WB. Recent studies of bodily effects of fear, rage and pain. In: Dennis W, editor. Readings in the History of Psychology. New York: Appleton; 1948. p. 482–4.
19. Selye H. Stress and disease. Science 1955;122:625–31.
20. Pavlov I. The relation of non conditioned reflex excitability and of conditioned reflex function in conditioned salivary reflexes. Kiscri Orvostud 1954 Non;6(6):549–56.
21. Ader R, Cohen N, Felten D. Psychoneuroimmunology: Interactions between the nervous system and the immune system. Lancet 1995;345(8942):99–103.
22. Cohen S, Herbert TB. Health psychology: Psychological factors and physical disease from the perspective of human psychoneuroimmunology. Annual Review of Psychology 1996;47:113–42.
23. Benson H, Beary JF, Carol MP. The relaxation response. Psychiatry 1974 Feb;37(1):37–46.
24. Kabat-Zinn J. An outpatient program in behavioral medicine for chronic pain patients based on the practice of mindfulness meditation: Theoretical considerations and preliminary results. General Hospital Psychiatry 1982 1982;4:33–47.
25. Wallace RK, Benson H, Wilson AF. A wakeful hypometabolic physiologic state. The American Journal of Physiology 1971 Sep;221(3):795–9.
26. Benson H, Lehmann JW, Malhotra MS, Goldman RF, Hopkins J, Epstein MD. Body temperature changes during the practice of g Tum-mo yoga. Nature 1982 Jan 21;295(5846):234–6.
27. Kabat-Zinn J. Full Catastrophe Living: Using the Wisdom of Your Body and Mind to Face Stress, Pain, and Illness. New York: Delacourt; 1990.
28. Kabat-Zinn J, Lipworth L, Burney R. The clinical use of mindfulness meditation for the self-regulation of chronic pain. Journal of Behavioral Medicine 1985 Jun;8(2):163–90.
29. Kabat-Zinn. Wherever you go, there you are: Mindfulness meditation in everyday life. New York: Hyperion; 1994.
30. Grossman P, Niemann L, Schmidt S, Walach H. Mindfulness-based stress reduction and health benefits. A meta-analysis. Journal of Psychosomatic Research 2004;57(1):35–43.
31. Ott MJ, Norris RL, Bauer-Wu SM. Mindfulness meditation for oncology patients: A discussion and critical review. Integrative Cancer Therapies 2006;5(2):98–108.
32. Blanchard CM, Denniston MM, Baker F, Ainsworth SR, Courneya KS, Hann DM, et al. Do adults change their lifestyle behaviors after a cancer diagnosis? American Journal of Health Behavior 2003 May–Jun;27(3):246–56.
33. Baider L, Uziely B, De-Nour AK. Progressive muscle relaxation and guided imagery in cancer patients. General Hospital Psychiatry 1994;16(5):340–7.
34. Sloman R. Relaxation and the relief of cancer pain. The Nursing Clinics of North America 1995;30(4):697–709.
35. Moskowitz L. Psychological management of postsurgical pain and patient adherence. Hand Clinics 1996;12(1):129–37.
36. Ross MC, Bohannon AS, Davis DC, Gurchiek L. The effects of a short-term exercise program on movement, pain, and mood in the elderly. Results of a pilot study. Journal of Holistic Nursing 1999;17(2):139–47.
37. Spiegel D. Psychosocial aspects of breast cancer treatment. Seminars in Oncology 1997;24(1):36–47.
38. Walker L, Walker M, Odston K. Psychological, clinical and pathological effects of relaxation training and guided imagery during chemotherapy. British Journal of Cancer 1999;80 (1–2):262–8.

39. Wallace KG. Analysis of recent literature concerning relaxation and imagery interventions for cancer pain. Cancer Nursing 1997;20(2):79–87.
40. Richardson MA, Post-White J, Grimm EA, Moye LA, Singletary SE, Justice B. Coping, life attitudes, and immune responses to imagery and group support after breast cancer treatment. Alternative Therapies in Health & Medicine 1997;3(5):62–70.
41. Turner-Cobb JM, Sephton SE, Koopman C, Blake-Mortimer J, Spiegel D. Social support and salivary cortisol in women with metastatic breast cancer. Psychosomatic Medicine 2000;62(3):337–45.
42. Coker KH. Meditation and prostate cancer: Integrating a mind/body intervention with traditional therapies. Seminars in Urologic Oncology 1999;17(2):111–8.
43. Massion AO, Teas J, Hebert JR, Wertheimer MD, Kabat-Zinn J. Meditation, melatonin and breast/prostate cancer: Hypothesis and preliminary data. Medical Hypotheses 1995;44(1):39–46.
44. Arakawa S. Relaxation to reduce nausea, vomiting, and anxiety induced by chemotherapy in Japanese patients. Cancer Nursing 1997;20(5):342–9.
45. Manyande A, Berg S, Gettins D, Stanford SC, Mazhero S, Marks DF. Preoperative rehearsal of active coping imagery influences subjective and hormonal responses to abdominal surgery. Psychosomatic Medicine 1995;57:177–82.
46. Syrjala KL, Chapko ME. Evidence for a biopsychosocial model of cancer treatment-related pain. Pain 1995;61(1):69–79.
47. Troesch LM, Rodehaver CB, Delaney EA, Yanes B. The influence of guided imagery on chemotherapy-related nausea and vomiting. Oncology Nursing Forum 1993;20(8):1179–85.
48. Fawzy FI, Fawzy NW, Arndt LA, Pasnau RO. Critical review of psychosocial interventions in cancer care. Archives of General Psychiatry 1995;52:100–13.
49. Helgeson VS, Cohen S, Schulz R, Yasko J. Group support interventions for women with breast cancer: Who benefits from what? Health Psychology 2000;19(2):107–14.
50. Spiegel D, Bloom JR, Yalom I. Group support for patients with metastatic cancer. A randomized outcome study. Archives of General Psychiatry 1981;38:527–33.
51. Fawzy FI, Cousins N, Fawzy NW, Kemeny ME, Elashoff R, Morton D. A structured psychiatric intervention for cancer patients: I. Changes over time in methods of coping and affective disturbance. Archives of General Psychiatry 1990;47:720–5.
52. Helgeson VS, Cohen S, Schulz R, Yasko J. Education and peer discussion group interventions and adjustment to breast cancer. Archives of General Psychiatry 1999;56(4):340–7.
53. Richardson JL, Shelton DR, Krailo M, Levine AM. The effect of compliance with treatment on survival among patients with hematologic malignancies. Journal of Clinical Oncology 1990;8:356–64.
54. Taimini I. The science of yoga: Madras: The Theosophical Publishing House; 1961.
55. Patanjali. Yoga Sutras. 800bc.
56. Rinpoche NN. Yantra Yoga. Arcidosso, Italy: Shang shung Edizioni; 1998.
57. Collins C. Yoga: intuition, preventive medicine, and treatment. Journal of Obstetric, Gynecologic, & Neonatal Nursing 1998;27(5):563–8.
58. Garfinkel M, Schumacher HR, Jr. Yoga. Rheumatic Diseases Clinics of North America 2000;26(1):125–32.
59. La Forge R. Mind-body fitness: Encouraging prospects for primary and secondary prevention. The Journal of Cardiovascular Nursing 1997;11(3):53–65.
60. Nagendra HR, Nagarathna R. Applications of integrated approach of yoga therapy – A review. A new life for asthmatics: Vivekananda Kendra; 1986.
61. Dostalek C, Faber J, Krasa H, Roldan E, Vele F. Yoga meditation effect on the EEG and EMG activity. Activitas Nervosa Superior 1979;21(1):41.
62. Dostalek C, Lepicovska V. Hathayoga–a method for prevention of cardiovascular diseases. Activitas Nervosa Superior 1982;Suppl 3(Pt 2):444–52.
63. Gode JD, Singh RH, Settiwar RM, Gode KD, Udupa KN. Increased urinary excretion of testosterone following a course of yoga in normal young volunteers. Indian Journal of Medical Sciences 1974;28(4–5):212–5.

64. Gopal K, Lakshmanan S. Some observations on Hatha Yoga: The bandhas: An anatomical study. Indian Journal of Medical Sciences 1972;26(9):564–74.
65. Grim PF. Psychotherapy by somatic alteration. Mental Hygiene 1969;53(3):451–8.
66. Stek RJ, Bass BA. Personal adjustment and perceived locus of control among students interested in meditation. Psychological Reports 1973;32(3):1019–22.
67. Udupa KN, Singh RH. The scientific basis of yoga. Journal of the Amercian Medical Association 1972;220(10):1365.
68. Vahia NS, Doongaji DR, Jeste DV, Ravindranath S, Kapoor SN, Ardhapurkar I. Psychophysiologic therapy based on the concepts of Patanjail. A new approach to the treatment of neurotic and psychosomatic disorders. American Journal of Psychotherapy 1973;27(4):557–65.
69. Garfinkel MS, Schumacher HR, Jr, Husain A, Levy M, Reshetar RA. Evaluation of a yoga based regimen for treatment of osteoarthritis of the hands. The Journal of Rheumatology 1994;21(12):2341–3.
70. Ramaratnam S, Sridharan K. Yoga for epilepsy. Cochrane Database of Systematic Reviews 2000(3):CD001524.
71. Vedanthan PK, Kesavalu LN, Murthy KC, Duvall K, Hall MJ, Baker S, et al. Clinical study of yoga techniques in university students with asthma: A controlled study. Allergy and Asthma Proceedings 1998;19(1):3–9.
72. Nagarathna R, Nagendra HR. Yoga for bronchial asthma: A controlled study. British Medical Journal (Clinical Research Edition) 1985;291(6502):1077–9.
73. Mahajan AS, Reddy KS, Sachdeva U. Lipid profile of coronary risk subjects following yogic lifestyle intervention. Indian Heart Journal 1999;51(1):37–40.
74. Murugesan R, Govindarajulu N, Bera TK. Effect of selected yogic practices on the management of hypertension. Indian Journal of Physiology and Pharmacology 2000;44(2):207–10.
75. Janakiramaiah N, Gangadhar BN, Naga Venkatesha Murthy PJ, Harish MG, Subbakrishna DK, Vedamurthachar A. Antidepressant efficacy of Sudarshan Kriya Yoga (SKY) in melancholia: A randomized comparison with electroconvulsive therapy (ECT) and imipramine. Journal of Affective Disorders 2000;57(1–3):255–9.
76. Dash M, Telles S. Yoga training and motor speed based on a finger tapping task. Indian Journal of Physiology and Pharmacology 1999;43(4):458–62.
77. Telles S, Hanumanthaiah BH, Nagarathna R, Nagendra HR. Plasticity of motor control systems demonstrated by yoga training. Indian Journal of Physiology and Pharmacology 1994;38(2):143–4.
78. Malathi A, Damodaran A, Shah N, Patil N, Maratha S. Effect of yogic practices on subjective well being. Indian Journal of Physiology and Pharmacology 2000;44(2):202–6.
79. Malathi A, Damodaran A. Stress due to exams in medical students-role of yoga. Indian Journal of Physiology and Pharmacology 1999;43(2):218–24.
80. Telles S, Reddy SK, Nagendra HR. Oxygen consumption and respiration following two yoga relaxation techniques. Applied Psychophysiology and Biofeedback 2000;25(4):221–7.
81. Telles S, Nagarathna R, Nagendra HR, Desiraju T. Alterations in auditory middle latency evoked potentials during meditation on a meaningful symbol–"Om". The International Journal of Neuroscience 1994;76(1–2):87–93.
82. Telles S, Nagarathna R, Nagendra HR. Breathing through a particular nostril can alter metabolism and autonomic activities. Indian Journal of Physiology and Pharmacology 1994;38(2):133–7.
83. Telles S, Desiraju T. Recording of auditory middle latency evoked potentials during the practice of meditation with the syllable 'OM'. The Indian Journal of Medical Research 1993;98:237–9.
84. Telles S, Desiraju T. Heart rate and respiratory changes accompanying yogic conditions of single thought and thoughtless states. Indian Journal of Physiology and Pharmacology 1992;36(4):293–4.
85. Joseph CD. Psychological supportive therapy for cancer patients. Indian Journal of Cancer 1983;20(5):268–70.
86. Schwidurski-Maib G, Jochheim KA. Current status of after-care cures in oncologic patients. Rehabilitation 1987;26(2):75–6.

87. Vivekananda S. Raja Yoga. Madras: Advaita Ashram; 1970.
88. Rahula W. What the Buddha Taught. New York, NY: Grove Press; 1974.
89. Santideva. A Guide to the Bodhisattva Way of Life (Bodhicaryavatara). Ithace, NY: Snow Lion Publications; 1997.
90. Alexander CN, Langer EJ, Newman RI, Chandler HM, Davies JL. Transcendental meditation, mindfulness, and longevity: An experimental study with the elderly. Journal of Personality and Social Psychology 1989 Dec;57(6):950–64.
91. Anderson DJ. Transcendental Meditation as an alternative to heroin abuse in servicemen. The American Journal of Psychiatry 1977 Nov;134(11):1308–9.
92. Eppley KR, Abrams AI, Shear J. Differential effects of relaxation techniques on trait anxiety: A meta-analysis. Journal of Clinical Psychology 1989 Nov;45(6):957–74.
93. Orme-Johnson D. Medical care utilization and the transcendental meditation program. Psychosomatic Medicine 1987 Sep–Oct;49(5):493–507.
94. Orme-Johnson D, Dillbeck MC, Wallace RK, Landrith GS, III. Intersubject EEG coherence: Is consciousness a field? The International Journal of Neuroscience 1982 May;16(3–4): 203–9.
95. Orme-Johnson D, Zimmerman E, Hawkins M. Maharishi's Vedic psychology: The science of the cosmic psyche. In: Kao KSR, Sinha D, editors. Asian Perspectives on Psychology. New Delhi: Sage Publications; 1997.
96. Orme-Johnson DW. Autonomic stability and transcendental meditation. Psychosomatic Medicine 1973 Jul–Aug;35(4):341–9.
97. US GPO. Alternative Medicine: Expanding Medical Horizons. A Report to the National Institutes of Health on Alternative Medical Systems and Practices in the United States, 1992; 1994.
98. Wallace RK. Physiological effects of transcendental meditation. Science 1970 Mar 27;167(926):1751–4.
99. Orme-Johnson DW, Schneider RH, Son YD, Nidich S, Cho ZH. Neuroimaging of meditation's effect on brain reactivity to pain. Neuroreport 2006 Aug 21;17(12):1359–63.
100. Tooley GA, Armstrong SM, Norman TR, Sali A. Acute increases in night-time plasma melatonin levels following a period of meditation. Biological Psychology 2000;53(1):69–78.
101. Kabat-Zinn J, Massion AO, Kristeller J, Peterson LG, Fletcher KE, Pbert L, et al. Effectiveness of a meditation-based stress reduction program in the treatment of anxiety disorders. The American Journal of Psychiatry 1992;149(7):936–43.
102. Kabat-Zinn J, Wheeler E, Light T, Skillings A, Scharf MJ, Cropley TG, et al. Influence of a mindfulness meditation-based stress reduction intervention on rates of skin clearing in patients with moderate to severe psoriasis undergoing phototherapy (UVB) and photochemotherapy (PUVA). Psychosomatic Medicine 1998;60(5):625–32.
103. Baer RA, Smith GT, Hopkins J, Krietemeyer J, Toney L. Using self-report assessment methods to explore facets of mindfulness. Assessment 2006;13(1):27–45.
104. Davidson RJ, Kabat-Zinn J, Schumacher J, Rosenkranz M, Muller D, Santorelli SF, et al. Alterations in brain and immune function produced by mindfulness meditation. Psychosomatic Medicine 2003 Jul–Aug;65(4):564–70.
105. Davidson RJ. Affective style, psychopathology, and resilience: Brain mechanisms and plasticity. The American Psychologist 2000 Nov;55(11):1196–214.
106. Davidson RJ. Emotion and affective style: Hemisphere substrates. Psychological Science 1992;3:39–43.
107. Davidson RJ, Ekman P, Saron CD, Senulis JA, Friesen WV. Approach-withdrawal and cerebral asymmetry: Emotional expression and brain physiology. I. Journal of Personality and Social Psychology 1990 Feb;58(2):330–41.
108. Lutz A, Greischar LL, Rawlings NB, Ricard M, Davidson RJ. Long-term meditators self-induce high-amplitude gamma synchrony during mental practice. Proceedings of the National Academy of Sciences of the United States of America 2004 Nov 16;101(46): 16369–73.

109. Fries P, Reynolds JH, Rorie AE, Desimone R. Modulation of oscillatory neuronal synchronization by selective visual attention. Science 2001 Feb 23;291(5508):1560–3.
110. Miltner WH, Braun C, Arnold M, Witte H, Taub E. Coherence of gamma-band EEG activity as a basis for associative learning. Nature 1999 Feb 4;397(6718):434–6.
111. Srinivasan R, Russell DP, Edelman GM, Tononi G. Increased synchronization of neuromagnetic responses during conscious perception. The Journal of Neuroscience 1999 Jul 1;19(13):5435–48.
112. Tallon-Baudry C, Bertrand O, Peronnet F, Pernier J. Induced gamma-band activity during the delay of a visual short-term memory task in humans. The Journal of Neuroscience 1998 Jun 1;18(11):4244–54.
113. Teasdale JD, Segal ZV, Williams JM, Ridgeway VA, Soulsby JM, Lau MA. Prevention of relapse/recurrence in major depression by mindfulness-based cognitive therapy. Journal of Consulting and Clinical Psychology 2000;68(4):615–23.
114. Teasdale JD, Moore RG, Hayhurst H, Pope M, Williams S, Segal ZV. Metacognitive awareness and prevention of relapse in depression: Empirical evidence. Journal of Consulting and Clinical Psychology 2002;70(2):275–87.
115. Speca M, Carlson LE, Goodey E, Angen M. A randomized, wait-list controlled clinical trial: The effect of a mindfulness meditation-based stress reduction program on mood and symptoms of stress in cancer outpatients. Psychosomatic Medicine 2000;62(5):613–22.
116. Carlson LE, Ursuliak Z, Goodey E, Angen M, Speca M. The effects of a mindfulness meditation-based stress reduction program on mood and symptoms of stress in cancer outpatients: 6-month follow-up. Supportive Care in Cancer 2001;9(2):112–23.
117. Carlson LE, Garland SN. Impact of mindfulness-based stress reduction (MBSR) on sleep, mood, stress and fatigue symptoms in cancer outpatients. International Journal of Behavioral Medicine 2005;12(4):278–85.
118. Johnson JA. Chinese medical Qigong therapy: A comprehensive clinical guide. 1st ed: International Institute of Medical Qigong; 2000.
119. Jonas W, Crawford C. Healing, intention, and energy medicine: Science, research methods, and clinical implications. 1st ed. New York: Churchill Livingstone; 2003.
120. Yang J-M. The Roots of Chinese Qigong. Secret for Health, Longevity, and Enlighment. Roslindale, MA: YMAA Publication Center; 1997.
121. Cohen KS. The Way of Qigong: The Art and Science of Chinese Energy Healing. New York: Ballentine Books; 1997.
122. Sancier KM. Therapeutic benefits of qigong exercises in combination with drugs. Journal of Alternative and Complementary Medicine (New York, N. Y.) 1999;5(4):383–9.
123. Wu W-H, Bandilla E, Ciccone DS, Yang J, Cheng S-CS, Carner N. Effects of qigong on late-stage complex regional pain syndrome. Alternative Therapies in Health and Medicine 1999;5(1):45–54.
124. Lee MS, Jang JW, Jang HS, Moon SR. Effects of Qi-therapy on blood pressure, pain and psychological symptoms in the elderly: A randomized controlled pilot trial. Complementary Therapies in Medicine 2003 Sep;11(3):159–64.
125. Li M, Chen K, Mo Z. Use of qigong therapy in the detoxification of heroin addicts. Alternative Therapies in Health and Medicine 2002 Jan-Feb;8(1):50–4, 6–9.
126. Lee MS, Huh HJ, Hong SS, Jang HS, Ryu H, Lee HS, et al. Psychoneuroimmunological effects of Qi-therapy: Preliminary study on the changes of level of anxiety, mood, cortisol and melatonin and cellular function of neutrophil and natural killer cells. Stress and Health 2001 Jan;17(1):17–24.
127. Hartman C, Manos T, Winter C, Hartman D, Li B, Smith J. Effects of T'ai Chi training on function and quality of life indicators in older adults with osteoarthritis. Journal of the American Geriatrics Society 2000 Dec;48(12):1553–9.
128. Li F, Fisher KJ, Weimer C, Shirai M. The Effects of Tai Chi training on self-rated sleep quality in older adults: A randomized controlled trial. Sleep 2003;26(Abstract Supplement):A423–4.

129. Tsai JC, Wang WH, Chan P, Lin LJ, Wang CH, Tomlinson B, et al. The beneficial effects of Tai Chi Chuan on blood pressure and lipid profile and anxiety status in a randomized controlled trial. Journal of Alternative and Complementary Medicine 2003 Oct;9(5):747–54.
130. Lee MS, Kim HJ, Moon SR. Qigong reduced blood pressure and catecholamine levels of patients with essential hypertension. International Journal of Neuroscience 2003 Dec;113(12):1691–701.
131. Ryu H, Jun CD, Lee BS, Choi BM, Kim HM, Chung HT. Effect of Qigong training on proportions of T-lymphocyte subsets in human peripheral-blood. The American Journal of Chinese Medicine 1995;23(1):27–36.
132. Lee MS, Jeong SM, Kim YK, Park KW, Ryu H, Moon SR. Qi-training enhances respiratory burst function and adhesive capacity of neutrophils in young adults: A preliminary study. The American Journal of Chinese Medicine 2003;31(1):141–8.
133. Jones BM. Changes in cytokine production in healthy subjects practicing Guolin Qigong: A pilot study. BMC Complementary and Alternative Medicine 2001,1(1):8.
134. Wang C, Xu D. Influence of qigong therapy upon serum HDL-C in hypertensive patients. Chung Hsi i Chieh Ho Tsa Chih Chinese Journal of Modern Developments in Traditional Medicine 1989 Sep;9(9):435–544.
135. Li F, Harmer P, McAuley E, Duncan T, Duncan S, Chaumeton N, et al. An evaluation of the effects of Tai Chi exercise on physical function among older persons: A randomized controlled trial. Annals of Behavioral Medicine 2001;23(2):139–46.
136. Irwin MR, Pike JL, Cole JC, Oxman MN. Effects of a behavioral intervention, Tai Chi Chuan, on varicella-zoster virus specific immunity and health functioning in older adults. Psychosomatic Medicine 2003 Sep–Oct;65(5):824–30.
137. Lim YA, Boone T, Flarity JR, Thompson WR. Effects of Qigong on cardiorespiratory changes – a preliminary study. The American Journal of Chinese Medicine 1993;21(1):1–6.
138. Liang YJ, Cai YY, Wang ZX. The effects of Chinese traditional breathing training on the exercise test, resistance breathing and quality of life in chronic obstructive pulmonary disease patients. Chinese Medical Journal 1998 Apr;111(4):318.
139. Lai JS, Lan C, Wong MK, Teng SH. 2-Year trends in cardiorespiratory function among older Tai-Chi-Chuan practitioners and sedentary subjects. Journal of the American Geriatrics Society 1995 Nov;43(11):1222–7.
140. Mustian KM, Katula JA, Gill DL, Roscoe JA, Lang D, Murphy K. Tai Chi Chuan, health-related quality of life and self-esteem: A randomized trial with breast cancer survivors. Supportive Care in Cancer 2004 Dec;12(12):871–6.
141. Mustian KM, Katula JA, Zhao H. A pilot study to assess the influence of tai chi chuan on functional capacity among breast cancer survivors. The Journal of Supportive Oncology 2006 Mar;4(3):139–45.
142. Cohen L, Warneke C, Fouladi RT, Rodriguez MA, Chaoul-Reich A. Psychological adjustment and sleep quality in a randomized trial of the effects of a Tibetan yoga intervention in patients with lymphoma. Cancer 2004;100(10):2253–60.
143. Cohen L, Thornton B, Perkins G, Chandwani K, Sterner J, Chaoul-Reich A. A randomized trial of a Tibetan yoga intervention for breast cancer patients. Psychosomatic Medicine 2005;67(1):A33.
144. Nagendra HR, Nagarathna R. An integrated approach of yoga therapy for bronchial asthma: A 3-54-month prospective study. The Journal of Asthma 1986;23(3):123–37.
145. Cohen L, Chandwani KD, Thornton B, Perkins GH, Rivera E, Arun B, et al. Randomized trial of yoga in women with breast cancer undergoing radiation treatment. ASCO Annual Meeting Proceedings Part I Abstract no. 8505. Journal of Clinical Oncology 2006; 24:18S.
146. Antoni MH, Lutgendorf SK, Cole SW, Dhabhar FS, Sephton SE, McDonald PG, et al. The influence of bio-behavioural factors on tumour biology: Pathways and mechanisms. Nature Reviews. Cancer 2006;6(3):240–8.
147. Glaser R, Kiecolt-Glaser JK. Stress-induced immune dysfunction: Implications for health. Nature Reviews. Immunology 2005;5(3):243–51.

Chapter 11
Herbs and Other Botanicals: Interactions with Pharmaceuticals

Jyothirmai Gubili, Simon Yeung, and Barrie Cassileth

Contents

11.1 Introduction 161
11.2 Definitions 162
11.3 Cancer Patient Use of Herbal Supplements 162
11.4 Botanicals Research 163
References 176

Abstract Herbal supplements are being used by an increasing number of cancer patients for symptom relief both during and after treatment. But botanicals contain biologically active compounds that can interfere with chemotherapeutic drugs and other medications. Research is underway to determine the mechanism of action and beneficial effects of botanicals.

Keywords: Cancer · symptom management · herbal supplements · botanicals research.

11.1 Introduction

Herbal supplements are popular in the United States, and their use has increased over the last three decades. According to the National Health Interview Survey conducted by the Centers for Disease Control and Prevention in 2002, nearly 12% (38 million) Americans use botanicals [1]. The use of herbs is prevalent among cancer patients, especially those with breast cancer [2], prostate cancer [3], head and neck cancers [4], and pediatric cancers [5, 6].

J. Gubili
Memorial Sloan-Kettering Cancer Center, 1429 First Avenue, New York, NY 10021
e-mail: gubilij@mskcc.org

However, herb–drug interactions remain a serious potential concern, as few botanicals have been studied in humans to rule out such interactions [7, 8]. In this chapter, we present information on herbs and herbal agents, especially those used by cancer patients. The general use of herbs and herbal compounds is reviewed. Selected research conducted in our department is described, including studies of Huanglian, Jin fu kang, Maitake, and Sho-saiko-to (SST).

11.2 Definitions

Botanicals, also known as Phytomedicinals, are derived from plants, although algae, mushrooms, and other edible fungi also fall into this category. Phytomedicinals may contain the whole plant or its leaves, flowers, fruits, seeds, stem, wood, bark, roots, rhizomes, or exudates. The plant's fresh juices, gums, fixed oils, essential oils, resins, and dry powders also are used. Often two or more botanicals are combined to increase potency as in traditional Chinese medicine. Excipients may be added to stabilize active components or enhance the overall effect. The final products may take the form of powder, liquid, pills, or topical preparations.

11.3 Cancer Patient Use of Herbal Supplements

Many cancer patients use herbal supplements as an adjunct to chemotherapy or other cancer treatment to alleviate symptoms both during and after treatment. Conventional management of cancer-related symptoms typically involves use of pharmaceuticals. However, many are not very effective or are associated with adverse effects. For example, use of ondansetron and dexamethasone is only moderately beneficial against pre-chemotherapy ("anticipatory") nausea, which affects about one in three patients, and against low-grade nausea that persists for several days after chemotherapy [9, 10]. Benzodiazepines, commonly prescribed for treating insomnia, can affect the central nervous system [11]. In addition, prolonged use of drugs may lead to dependence. These concerns along with cost of conventional medications have led increasing numbers of cancer patients to seek herbal remedies for symptom relief.

But even though herbal products are perceived as being safe and natural, they contain biologically active compounds that can interfere with the action of chemotherapeutic drugs and other prescription medications. The popular herb St. John's wort is used to treat moderate to severe depression [12], but several adverse effects have been reported from its use that include dizziness, nausea, fatigue, and headaches. It also induces cytochrome P450 3A4, an enzyme responsible for metabolism of several drugs, including those used during chemotherapy [13]. Another major concern is the lack of information about herb–drug interactions for many other commonly used herbs. This has led to an increase in research efforts to determine the mechanism of action and beneficial effects of botanicals.

However, the problems in conducting botanicals research are, first, it is difficult to secure a patent for a natural substance. Pharmaceutical companies that spend the most money to support research are reluctant to invest funds and resources on products that do not ensure substantial financial return. Second, unlike synthetic pharmaceuticals, where a standard drug and dose regimen can be used for all patients, herbalists usually customize botanicals based on the individual's condition. This approach makes it difficult to establish a dose range and study the interactions. Third, the properties of botanicals may vary between batches, complicating standardization, and the study of biological effects. It is also difficult to obtain Food and Drug Administration (FDA) approval for use of a variety of formulations in a single study. Fortunately, in the recent years, the National Institutes of Health (NIH) has begun sponsoring high quality botanicals research [14].

11.4 Botanicals Research

11.4.1 Huanglian—A Phase I Study of the Chinese Herb Huanglian (Coptis chinensis) in Patients with Advanced Solid Tumors

11.4.1.1 Background

Huanglian (*C. chinensis*) is an herb that has been widely used in China for several thousand years. It was first described in the Divine Husbandman's Classic of the Materia Medica in the second century as a remedy to "clear heat, dry dampness, and to eliminate toxins". In traditional medicine, huanglian is used to treat diarrhea or dysentery. It is also often used in combination with other herbs in a decoction to treat inflammatory conditions ranging from gastroenteritis to acute febrile illnesses.

11.4.1.2 Research

Laboratory Studies

Modern scientific studies have confirmed some of huanglian's medicinal effects. In vitro studies have shown huanglian can suppress the growth of *Heliobacter pylori* and the intestinal parasite *Blastocystis hominis* [15–17]. It inhibits lipid peroxidation in rat tissues and has a protective effect against chemically induced diabetes in rats [18]. Other studies have explored its effect in treating burn wounds [19] and in inhibiting platelet aggregation [20].

The alkaloid berberine is thought to be the largest component constituting up to 25% of huanglian, but other components including coptisine, palmatine, jatrorrhizine, bauerenol, and epiberberine have been identified [21].

Some studies have also examined huanglian's anticancer properties. Extracts of huanglian have been shown to inhibit topoisomerase I to levels that are equivalent to that of camptothecins [22, 23]. Continuous exposure of HepG2 hepatoma cells to berberine inhibits tumor cell growth in a dose-dependent manner [24]. Oral administration of huanglian to laboratory rats inhibits the formation of azoxymethane-induced aberrant crypt foci, a putative pre-neoplastic lesion for colon cancer [25].

Huanglian is generally non-toxic. Dose as high as 27g/kg/day produced no toxicity in mice [26]. Huanglian has been administered to patients as an aqueous, herbal tea at doses of 20–30 g/day without toxicity.

Some data exists on the pharmacokinetics of huanglian. In rabbits, cats, rats, and mice, components of huanglian were absorbed rapidly through the upper gastrointestinal tract [27]. Oral administration of huanglian extract to laboratory rats resulted in serum levels of berberine measurable by high performance liquid chromatography (HPLC) [28].

Despite positive results, the role of huanglian as an anti-cancer drug has not been defined. It is possible that the number of components within huanglian may result in a broad-based inhibition of many cancer targets. Because berberine constitutes the major fraction of huanglian (25%), we also tested a 10 µg/ml solution of berberine to determine the degree to which it inhibited proliferation of the MKN-74 cells. Under the conditions tested, berberine was not able to inhibit cell proliferation to the same degree as either huanglian or its metabolites. This supports the hypothesis that the anti-tumor effects observed in vitro are due to other components present in the huanglian extract. This provides a rationale for clinical development of this agent as a whole herb in cancer therapy.

Laboratory studies showed that a water extract of huanglian inhibited the growth colony formation of human cancer cell lines MKN-74 (gastric, Panel A), HCT-116 (colon, Panel B), MCF-7 (breast, Panel C) and MDA468 (breast, Panel D). Additional studies showed that huanglian extract suppresses cdc2 kinase activity in association with loss of cyclin B1 protein, resulting in blocking the G2 phase of cell division.

11.4.1.3 Our Study

Aims and Endpoints

The current plan is to conduct a phase I clinical trial to determine a safe and effective optimal dose of huanglian for subsequent phase II trials. Classic phase I drug testing requires determining the maximum tolerated dose. Based on traditional use and animal data, high doses of huanglian can be consumed (up to 30 g) without toxicity [26]. Because toxic effects may not be seen, other endpoints such as biologic, molecular, and pharmacologic are used as surrogates in this study.

1. **Biologic:** A preclinical study showed that the metabolites of huanglian can inhibit cell growth in vitro. If the plasma from patients following administration of huanglian is added directly to the tumor cell lines resulting in a 50% or more inhibition of cell growth, a biologically active target dose is achieved.
2. **Molecular:** Huanglian suppresses cyclin B1, which suppresses the activity of cdc2 kinase. The same tumor cells that are exposed to the metabolites of huanglian for the biologic assays are used to make protein lysates for purposes of

determining cyclin B1 protein expression by western blot before and after drug therapy. A 50% suppression of cyclin B1 protein is the targeted molecular effect.
3. **Pharmacologic:** As berberine constitutes approximately 25% of the total huanglian extract, a pharmacologic endpoint is achieved when a predefined plasma berberine concentration is reached.

Dose escalation based on conventional toxicity assessment: Both conventional toxicities and surrogate markers of response will be assessed concurrently. The traditional toxicity escalation schedule is based on standard NCI toxicity criteria and a "surrogate response" dose escalation schedule which is based on biologic, molecular, and pharmacologic markers of activity, as determined in our preclinical laboratory studies. This latter schedule will be invoked in the absence of traditional toxicity. An algorithm determines the next dose level to be used based on data from both schedules.

Study Agent

In traditional Chinese medicine, huanglian is prepared by boiling in hot water followed by extraction of water soluble components. The study agent is made in a manner that mimics the traditional extraction method. Raw huanglian herb is heated in distilled water to 100°C for 1 h. The insoluble substances are removed and the remaining solution is boiled to dryness. The dry powder is then collected and formulated into standardized capsules for dispensing. This approach allows controlling the amount of botanical to be administered to patients.

The range of huanglian used in traditional Chinese medicine is 1.5–9 g/day. Thirty grams of raw herbs yields around 6 g (20%) of huanglian extract. A starting dose of 1 g will be comparable to that commonly used as a daily dose of 5 g.

The material for the study is prepared by an experienced current good manufacturing practice (cGMP) manufacturing facility under contract from Memorial Sloan-Kettering Cancer Center. The product contains berberine (as determined qualitatively and qualitatively by HPLC) $25\% \pm 5\%$ total weight. Heavy metals such as arsenic are within acceptable limits.

Subject Selection

The study is open to all patients with advanced solid tumors refractory to standard therapy. Patients who have uncontrolled infection, history of cardiac arrhythmias are excluded. Pregnant women and patients who are using antiseizure medication are also excluded due to potential adverse effects. All patients are registered through Memorial Sloan-Kettering Cancer Center. An estimated 20–30 patients will be needed for the trial. Pretreatment clinical assessments are performed within 14 days after recruitment. These include medical history, including medications taken during the month prior to enrollment, complete physical examination with neurologic exam, Karnofsky performance, blood test, EKG, tumor biopsy as well as confirmed malignancy. Baseline blood serum sample is obtained before starting treatment as control for subsequent surrogate marker determinations.

Treatment Plan

Patients receive capsules of the powdered extract of the huanglian root to be taken orally four times a day. Treatment continues until either progression of disease or detection of limiting toxicities. The number of capsules administered each day depends on the patient dose level.

11.4.2 Jin Fu Kang —Safety and Pharmacokinetic Study of Jin Fu Kang in Combination with Docetaxel for Patients with Non-Small Cell Lung Cancer.

11.4.2.1 Background

Despite advances in therapy and attempts at prevention through smoking cessation and improved treatment, lung cancer continues to be the leading cause of cancer deaths in the United States. The American Cancer Society estimated that 170,000 new cases will be diagnosed in the year 2006 with 160,000 deaths [29]. More Americans will die from lung cancer than any other cancer [30].

Approximately 80% of lung cancer patients have non-small cell lung cancer (NSCLC). For patients with early-stage disease, surgical resection is often the best option. However, more than three-quarters of patients present at diagnosis with locally advanced or disseminated disease that is not amenable to surgery [31], and many resected patients relapse and present with disseminated disease [32]. For patients with locally advanced or metastatic NSCLC, systemic chemotherapy is the mainstay of treatment.

There is some evidence that second-line chemotherapy may also be of benefit in NSCLC. In a trial of patients who progressed after platinum-based therapy, lower dose docetaxel was shown to increase survival compared to best supportive care alone; improvements in symptom scores and reduced use of medication to treat tumor related-symptoms were also reported [33]. The U.S. FDA has approved 3 weekly 75 mg/m^2 docetaxel for the treatment of patients with locally advanced or metastatic NSCLC after failure of prior chemotherapy.

Although it has been demonstrated that chemotherapy treatment is superior to best supportive care, and that newer agents and combinations lead to incremental increases in survival and quality of life, the overall picture remains extremely grim. Improvements in survival resulting from chemotherapy have been small: median survival for patients with advanced NSCLC remains under 1 year, with fewer than 5% of patients surviving more than 5 years [34].

Jin Fu Kang is an oral liquid containing extracts from 12 botanicals. It was initially developed as a treatment for lung cancer in the late 1960s at the Shanghai

University of Traditional Chinese Medicine. The formula was modified several times until it was finalized in 1991. A series of clinical trials were conducted between 1970 and 1997 with generally positive results. In 1999, the Chinese drug administration (SDA, equivalent of the US FDA) approved Jin Fu Kang as a class III new drug for the treatment of NSCLC in China. The manufacturer estimates that over 12,000 patients have been treated with Jin Fu Kang since 1992.

11.4.2.2 Research

Laboratory Studies

Some of Jin Fu Kang's constituents have been demonstrated to have anticancer activity in modern laboratory studies. Astragalus membranaceus is known to have immune stimulant effects that are pertinent to cancer. Extracts of Astragalus have been demonstrated to lead to a 10-fold potentiation of interleukin (IL)-2-generated lymphokine-activated killer cell cytotoxicity against murine renal cell cancer in vitro. This activity was retained in vivo, with Astragalus curing over 50% of BALB/c mice transplanted intraperitoneally with $1-2 \times 10^5$ syngeneic renal cancer cells [35]. Astragalus has been also reported to inhibit the development of spontaneous mammary tumorigenesis in SHN mice and again an immune mechanism has been implicated [36]. Immune stimulant effects have also been demonstrated in cancer patients. Using the local graft versus host (GVH) reaction as a test assay for T-cell function, Sun et al. [37] demonstrated that Astragalus restored GVH in 9 of 10 cancer patients.

Human Studies

Three early clinical trials of Jin Fu Kang conducted between 1970 and 1990 have been reported in brief. In the first study, 310 cases of NSCLC were treated with an early version of Jin Fu Kang without chemotherapy. Seventy percent of patients in the study were stage III or IV. Survival rates of 43% at 1 year and 11% at 2 years were reported [38]. This was followed by a randomized trial that compared Jin Fu Kang to chemotherapy (mitomycin C, vincristine, and methotrexate) in the treatment of 122 patients with stage III or IV NCCLC. Median survival in those randomized to Jin Fu Kang was more than twice that of patients on chemotherapy. One-year survival on Jin Fu Kang was 67% compared to 33% on chemotherapy ($P = 0.0003$) [39]. The trial was repeated including only adenocarcinoma patients ($n = 304$). The difference in median survival between Jin Fu Kang and chemotherapy was smaller (approximately a 50% increase in median survival) but still highly significant: survival rates at 1 year were 61% on Jin Fu Kang compared to 37% on chemotherapy ($P < 0.00005$) [40].

In the first randomized trial using the final formula of Jin Fu Kang, 271 patients with unresectable NSCLC were randomized to receive Jin Fu Kang, chemotherapy, or both in a ratio of 2:1:1.5. Chemotherapy consisted of cisplatin, mitomycin c, and doxorubicin (MAP). Response rates were 11, 11, and 21% in the Jin Fu Kang, chemotherapy and combined groups, respectively. Although this difference in response was not statistically significant ($P = 0.1$ comparing chemotherapy to combination), 1-year survival was significantly higher in Jin Fu Kang and combination treatment than in the group receiving chemotherapy alone (76.4, 72.5, and 43.8%). Clinical response, evaluated by Karnofsky performance status and weight gain, was superior in both groups receiving Jin Fu Kang. Sixty percent of patients lost weight during chemotherapy compared to only 20% of those on combination therapy ($P = 0.001$). Differences were also reported in immunologic endpoints [41, 42].

The final trial, and the one considered pivotal by the SDA, accrued 290 patients with unresectable NSCLC from three hospitals. In keeping with previous studies, patients were randomized to Jin Fu Kang, chemotherapy, or both. Patients in the two chemotherapy arms received either cyclophosphamide, doxorubicin, and cisplatin, or mitomycin C, vindesine, or cisplatin. Weight loss was again much more common during chemotherapy treatment than combination therapy (59 versus 21%; $P < 0.0005$). There was certainly no indication of an increase in toxicity by adding Jin Fu Kang to chemotherapy; indeed, rates of certain toxicities such as neutropenia were lower in Jin Fu Kang plus chemotherapy compared to chemotherapy alone (34 versus 57%; $P = 0.0006$) [43].

A recent meta-analysis found Astragalus-based Chinese herbal medicine, such as Jin Fu Kang, may increase effectiveness of platinum-based chemotherapy [44].

In the Chinese trials, no serious adverse events were reported for single agent Jin Fu Kang. Moreover, rates of toxicity were lower in the Jin Fu Kang plus chemotherapy group than in patients treated with chemotherapy alone. Animal studies suggest Jin Fu Kang has low toxicity.

Our Study

The results of the above studies are sufficiently provocative to warrant further research, especially given the very poor prognosis and limited treatment options for this patient group. There is empirical evidence that Jin Fu Kang potentiates the effects of conventional cytotoxic agents. We are conducting a trial in order to establish tolerability and safety in a U.S. setting and provide preliminary data on treatment efficacy.

Study Agent

The Jin Fu Kang is supplied by Jianxi Yicun Pharmaceutical Company in China in liquid form in 10-ml vials, which is self-administered orally by patients. MSKCC has obtained an IND for Jin Fu Kang. The extraction method is cold percolation, and the techniques follow those of the Chinese pharmacopeia. Jin Fu Kang is subject to rigorous quality control to ensure that the product is not adulterated with potent, toxic, or addictive botanical substances, synthetic or highly purified drugs, or biotechnology derived or other naturally derived drugs.

The quality standards for Jin Fu Kang can be determined by identifying the four major component botanicals, Huang Qi (*Astragalus membranaceus*), Shan Zhu Yu (*Cornus officinalis*), Nu Zhen Zi (*Ligustri lucidum*), and Yin Yang Huo (*Epimedium sagittatum*) using Thin Layer Chromatography. Batch consistency is based on the standardized content of Icariin. Icariin is a glycoside present in one of the ingredients, Yin Yang Huo (*Epimedium sagittatum*). This constituent can be detected qualitatively and quantitatively by HPLC. The manufacturer has determined and selected Icariin as a marker for quality evaluation assay. Official standard states that Jin Fu Kang should contain no less than 1 mg of Icariin per 10 ml. An independent lab in the United States conducts quality tests on this product before it is administered to patients.

The traditional first step in a study of an anticancer agent would be to conduct a dose-finding phase I study. We do not feel that a phase I trial of Jin Fu Kang is indicated because the Chinese data have provided evidence of a safe and effective dose. We therefore designed a study using a combination of Jin Fu Kang with docetaxel in patients with NSCLC who do not respond to standard therapy or in those without any treatment options. The aim is to determine the toxicity of Jin Fu Kang/docetaxel combination and to determine whether Jin Fu Kang affects the pharmacokinetics of docetaxel and to provide preliminary efficacy and survival data.

Inclusion Criteria

Patients included in this study must have confirmed stage III or IV NSCLC, and docetaxel therapy for cancer is clinically indicated. Patients who have pancytopenia and compromised liver function are excluded. Other inclusion and exclusion criteria also apply per MSKCC policy.

Recruitment Plan

All patients at MSKCC who meet the inclusion criteria are identified at the time of clinical evaluation of chemotherapy. Because Jin Fu Kang treatment is likely to have high patient acceptability, our target is to accrue 20 patients in the course of 12–18 months.

Pretreatment evaluation, including complete medical history, physical examination, complete blood count (CBC), and so on, will be performed within 21 days prior to beginning of study.

Treatment/Intervention

Following traditional use, Jin Fu Kang is given on a 28-day cycle with a 3-day rest period between cycles. Docetaxel ($35\,mg/m^2$) is administered on days 1, 8, and 15 every 28 days.

Jin Fu Kang therapy starts on day 4, approximately 72 h after the first docetaxel dose, when plasma levels of docetaxel will be near zero. Blood samples for pharmacokinetic studies will be collected for the first and third doses of docetaxel. Compliance with Jin Fu Kang will be assessed by asking patients to complete a daily diary for as long as they are taking the study botanical. Patients are withdrawn from study if they experience unacceptable toxicity; if they have progression of disease or start a cytotoxic chemotherapy agent other than docetaxel; or if the patient declines further treatment. Patients who continue treatment with Jin Fu Kang after two cycles of docetaxel will be monitored by their physician every 14 days.

At the time a patient is discontinued from protocol participation, physical exam, performance status, weight, hematology, chemistry, and response will be documented. Any adverse events that are considered possibly, probably, or definitely related to study drug will be followed until resolution. The patient or the patient's local physician will be contacted for such follow-up information.

11.4.3 Maitake—A Phase I/II study of Maitake Extract in Breast cancer Patients

11.4.3.1 Background

Despite advances in treatment of breast cancer, the American Cancer Society estimated that there will be 212,920 cases of invasive breast cancer and 40,970 deaths among women in the United States in 2006 [45]. Treatment options for breast cancer patients include surgery, radiotherapy, chemotherapy, and hormonal therapy. In addition, many patients take botanical supplements during treatment, usually in hopes of survival [46]. Although some herbals are known to have effects against breast cancer in vitro [47–49], there is very little information about their safety and efficacy. But with increase in use of herbal medicine, there is also a growing emphasis on clinical studies on botanicals.

Maitake *(Grifola frondosa)* is a giant edible mushroom grown in northeastern Japan. It can also be found in temperate forests in northeastern America where it is known as "hen of the woods" or "sheep's head." It is traditionally consumed raw, cooked, or as a tea. Besides being consumed as food, Maitake has been used in conjunction with chemotherapy to treat cancer in Asia. The commercially available form is a fractionated extract known as "D-fraction" or "MD-fraction" originally developed by the Japanese mycologist Dr. Hiroaki Nanba. The product is extracted from the fruit bodies of Maitake mushroom. It consists of beta-glucan (a polysaccharide with beta-1,6-linked main chain and 1,3-linked branches).

11.4.3.2 Research

Laboratory Studies

Although little is known about its mechanism of action, Maitake is thought to activate the immune system. Maitake extract has no apparent direct cytocidal activity [50, 51] and seems to act by host-mediated action. It potentiates the cytotoxicity of natural killer cells [52] and activates macrophages [51,53]. Maitake extracts also enhance T cell activities [51] and antibody response [54]. Other studies have shown Maitake to increase the weight and number of nucleated cells in the spleen and to activate alternative complement pathway [54].

Maitake also reverses suppression of macrophage, T cell, natural killer cell, and lymphocyte activity induced by N-butyl-N-butanolnitrosoamine in mice [55].

Other studies show that Maitake extract increases interferon (IFN)-γ production in CD4+ T cells, while reducing the production of IL-4. It also increased the production of IL-12p70 and IFN-gamma by antigen-presenting cells [56]. Transfer of dendritic cells from tumor-bearing mice that had been treated with Maitake extract protected the recipient mice against tumor implantation, suggesting a role for Maitake in modulating antigen presentation [57].

Human Studies

In a non randomized clinical study, the D-fraction was tested in 165 cancer patients with advanced breast, lung, or liver cancer. Patients received either Maitake D-fraction tablets with chemotherapy or Maitake D-fraction alone. Tumor regression or significant symptom improvements were observed in at least 50% of patients without significant side effects. The data suggest that Maitake D-fraction has a synergistic effect with chemotherapy. It appears also to ameliorate the side effects from chemotherapy [58].

Another study involved a total of 36 patients with advanced cancer who could not tolerate the side effects of standard treatments. They were given MD-fraction tablets and whole Maitake powder after discontinuing chemotherapy. Cancer regression or significant symptom improvements were observed in more than half of the patients. The authors concluded that Maitake may have the potential to reduce the size of lung, liver, and breast tumors. There were no adverse effects reported [59].

Our Study

Our previous lab studies showed that the MD-fraction of maitake significantly enhanced CFU-GM and increased bone marrow cell viability [60]. We have been studying the effects of a purified Maitake extract designed to determine dose–response relationships and to evaluate specificity of action. This is followed by a phase I/II dose escalation trial. The objectives of this study are to determine biological markers of immune response, which are altered by oral administration of Maitake; to determine dose-response of Maitake on immune function; and to confirm the safety of Maitake in humans.

Study Agent

The Maitake extract used for this study is extracted from the raw mushrooms provided by Yukiguni Maitake Co., Ltd., through the Tradeworks Group. Maitake are cultivated in an artifical setting with strict control over temperature, humidity, illumination, ventilation, and other environmental variables. This minimizes batch-to-batch variation of the product. The extract is formulated in glycerin and supplied as a liquid for oral administration.

Inclusion Criteria

Stage I, II, and III breast cancer patients who have undergone resection and are currently free of disease will be included in the study. These patients are relatively healthy, and therefore able to mount an adequate immune response to stimulants. Patients who have second primary malignancy, who have cancer therapy in the last 3 months, and who have history of autoimmune disease are excluded.

Recruitment Plan

Potential research subjects are identified by a member of the patient's treatment team or protocol investigators. Six subjects will be entered sequentially into one of four cohorts treated at increasing doses. A total of 24 patients will be recruited. Patients have the routine blood work involving CBC. A double baseline measurement of immune function is undertaken 1 week before the first dose and on day 0, prior to the first dose.

Treatment/Intervention

All six subjects on a given dose will be enrolled before the next higher dose cohort is opened for accrual. The doses to be used are from 0.2 to 6 mg/kg/day.

CBC and the immune studies are repeated weekly for 3 weeks. Patients complete a compliance diary documenting each dose of Maitake.

Immunologic endpoints are chosen to test the host's key innate and adaptive immune functions. The effect on the overall hematopoietic system is tested by CBC and differentials. Quantitative analysis of each class of immune cells will be done by immunophenotyping. Antigen-specific immune responses are evaluated by ex vivo assays of intracellular cytokine production upon the challenge of specific antigens. Respiratory oxygen burst tests are used to determine the function of monocytes and neutrophils. Patients are discontinued from the study immediately, if any side effects grade 2 or above as defined in the NCI Common Terminology Criteria for Adverse Events are reported.

11.4.4 Sho-Saiko-To—Sho-Saiko-To for Patients with Chronic Hepatitis C Who are Intolerant to or Have Contraindication to Interferon-Based Therapy: A Phase II Study

11.4.4.1 Background

Infection with the hepatitis C virus (HCV) has become a significant public health problem in the United States in recent years. According to the World Health Organization, an estimated 170 million persons are currently infected with 4 million new cases reported each year (http://www.who.int/mediacentre/factsheets/fs164/en/). HCV is spread through direct blood contact. Intravenous-drug abusers are especially at risk. Hepatitis C infection is a major risk factor for hepatocellular carcinoma (HCC). A high proportion of patients with HCC have evidence of HCV infection, particularly in southern Europe and Japan where prevalence of HCV in HCC is up to 75% [61–63]. Currently, there is no vaccine available for HCV.

The standard drug treatment for chronic hepatitis C consists of IFN with ribavirin. One of the presumed benefits is that by reducing viral load and liver inflammation, treatment reduces the risk of cirrhosis and thus HCC. However, the efficacy of IFN-based therapy is suboptimal. After 48 weeks of combined therapy with three times weekly IFN and ribavirin, only approximately 40% of treated patients with HCV genotype 1 have a sustained virologic response [64,65]. Adverse effects, such as nausea, vomiting, anorexia, dizziness, dyspnea, insomnia, irritability, alopecia, rash, and pruritus, are frequently encountered during treatment [66]. IFN also causes leukopenia and occasionally thrombocytopenia, and the addition of ribavirin frequently leads to anemia with significant changes in hemoglobin. Many patients cannot tolerate the side effects from long-term treatment.

SST is a traditional botanical product from Japan that has been used to treat chronic liver disease. It based on an ancient Chinese herbal formula known as Xiao Chai Hu tang which contains a mixture of seven botanicals: Bupleurum root (*Bupleurum chinense*), Pinellia tuber (*Pinellia ternata*), Baical Skullcap root (*Scutellaria baicalensis*), Ginseng root (*Panax ginseng*), Licorice root (*Glycyrrhiza uralensis*), Ginger rhizome (*Zingiber officinale*), and Jujube fruit (*Zizyphus jujuba*). It may offer a new treatment option for patients with chronic hepatitis C who are intolerant to or who have a specific contraindication to IFN-based therapies.

11.4.4.2 Research

Laboratory Studies

In vitro research suggests SST, and its individual components may benefit patients who have hepatic fibrosis. Glycyrrhizin, a triterpenoid saponin extract found in licorice root, reduces serum aminotransferases [67]. Baicalein, a major flavonoid in Scutellaria, has antiproliferative and antifibrogenic effects when tested in hepatic stellate cells from rats [68]. Ginseng has been shown to inhibit the development of HCC in mice induced by diethylnitrosamine [69, 70], aflatoxin B1 [71], and a N-nitroso diethylamine and phenobarbital combination [72].

SST displayed inhibition of collagen formation, increased retinoid level, inhibited activation of Ito cells, and prevented liver fibrosis in rats [73–75]. It also has immune modulating effects. SST can induce production of IL-1β, IL-6, IFN-γ, tumor necrosis factor-α, and granulocyte-macrophage colony-stimulating factor [76,77].

SST was also shown to prevent liver injury and promote liver regeneration in animals. Rats treated with SST showed less fibrosis as indicated by reduced liver hydroxyproline and a smaller increase in serum hyaluronic acid as compared to the control group [78]. Moreover, SST-treated rats developed fewer preneoplastic lesions. Similar findings have been reported using carbon tetrachloride [75, 79] and N-nitroso morpholine [80] models of liver injury.

Human Studies

Several controlled and single-arm studies of SST have been conducted in hepatitis patients. In 1980s, a randomized trial was conducted in Japan. Two hundred and twenty-two patients with chronic active hepatitis B received either SST or placebo for 12 weeks. There were statistically significant differences between groups in aspartate transaminase and alanine transaminase. There was also an increase in anti-Hbe antibody during treatment in the SST but not in the placebo group [81].

In another trial, 93 patients with chronic hepatitis took SST for 36 months. Type III procollagen and 7S collagen values were reduced after 6 months, but there was no effect on serum laminin P1. Levels of glutamic pyruvate transaminase fell, but only after long-term treatment.

There is also evidence that SST might benefit hepatitis patients by preventing progression to HCC. A large prospective study was conducted in Japan [82]. Two hundred and sixty patients with cirrhosis were randomized by age, sex, hepatitis B antigen status, and liver function to treatment with SST or control. Patients were followed for 5 years with bimonthly alpha-fetoprotein measurements and quarterly ultrasonography. SST led to a one-third reduction in the incidence of HCC (23 versus 34%) and 40% reduction in deaths (24 versus 40%) as compared to control.

Adverse events associated with the consumption of SST have been reported in the literature. In an analysis of the manufacturers' drug monitoring system, SST-related pneumonitis was reported in 74 patients (approximately 1 in 20,000) leading to eight deaths [83]. Poorer outcome was associated with underlying lung disease and with continuing to take SST after the onset of pneumonitis.

Our Study

There is sufficient clinical, pharmacokinetic, and laboratory data with SST to warrant a phase II study. The objectives are to determine the effects of SST on hepatic injury in patients with chronic hepatitis C and to determine the effects of SST therapy on liver function and viral load. Liver injury is evaluated by histologic examination of liver biopsies taken prior to and following 52 weeks of SST therapy.

Study Agent

The SST study agent is provided by Honso, USA. The drug is prepared as a powder packed in sachets. It can be swallowed dry or dissolved in warm water. The product is manufactured according to cGMP and is subject to analysis for consistency. Each 2.5-g sachet is standardized to contain a predefined amount of marker compounds including baicalin, glycyrrhizin, and saikosaponin as identified by HPLC. Heavy metals and arsenic are tested to ensure that they are within the acceptable limits.

Inclusion Criteria

Patients with chronic hepatitis C, positive for HCV RNA by polymerase chain reaction (PCR), with elevated aminotransferases, who are intolerant to, or have a specific contraindication to IFN-based therapy are eligible for the study.

Exclusion Criteria

Patient coinfected with hepatitis B and HIV, has poor pulmonary function, use IFN and SST before, and has history of malignancy are excluded. Alcoholics, pregnant women are also excluded.

Recruitment Plan

Patients are identified at the time of clinical evaluation. A total of 30 patients treated with IFN-based therapy will be accrued.

Treatment/Intervention

All patients receive a liver biopsy before starting SST therapy. SST is given orally at a dose of 2.5 g three times a day for 52 weeks. A second liver biopsy will be performed for comparison at the end of 52 weeks. Blinded biopsies are evaluated by a histopathologist and scored according to the Knodell's histology activity index (HAI) for degree of hepatic inflammation and fibrosis [84]. Secondary outcomes, including change in aminotransferases and HCV viral load, are measured.

Clinical follow-up occurs every 3 months for 1 year. Patients are assessed for compliance and asked about side effects and pulmonary symptoms. At each clinic visit, a comprehensive metabolic profile is performed. At the 6-month clinic visit, a CBC is performed. At the 12-month clinic visit, quantitative HCV-RNA by PCR is obtained. Within 4 weeks after the 12-month clinic visit (after 52 weeks of SST therapy), the second liver biopsy is scheduled and performed.

11.4.5 Problems Associated with Botanicals Research

11.4.5.1 Standardization

One of the primary concerns in the development of botanical drugs is that of standardization and quality assurance. Unlike a pharmaceutical, which contains a single, chemically synthesized compound, botanical medicines contain a variety of different compounds. The concentration of each of these compounds can vary depending on where the plant was grown, moisture, temperature, and time of harvesting. This can inadvertently affect the biological activities of the final product. To ensure consistent quality and ingredients among batches, methods to standardize study preparations must be developed. For the identification and quality control, the presence and concentration of the most abundant active constituents is assayed.

Where active components are unknown, a surrogate chemical marker is used. A standardized botanical product must contain a predetermined amount of this marker in every batch.

11.4.5.2 Contaminants

Many contaminants such as pesticides, heavy metals, microbials, and extraneous matter are found in botanical preparations. Although most commercial herb farms use only approved pesticides, high amount of residual pesticides may be harmful. Heavy metals such as lead, mercury, and arsenic often appear in botanicals grown in soil with high concentrations of these metals naturally or as a result of industrial runoff. Such products are unsafe for consumption, especially by young children and pregnant women.

Botanical products are exposed to microbials during cultivation, handling, or storage. Pathogenic organisms in the final product as a result of improper cleaning could be detrimental if present.

References

1. CDC. *National Health Interview Survey.* 2002 [cited 2006 November 14]; Available from: http://wonder.cdc.gov/wonder/sci_data/surveys/nhis/type_txt/nhis2002/NHIS2002.asp.
2. Morris KT, Johnson N, Homer L, et al. A comparison of complementary therapy use between breast cancer patients and patients with other primary tumor sites. *Am J Surg* 2000;179(5):407–11.
3. Lippert MC, McClain R, Boyd JC, et al. Alternative medicine use in patients with localized prostate carcinoma treated with curative intent. *Cancer* 1999;86(12):2642–8.
4. Gurley BJ, Gardner SF, Hubbard MA. Content versus label claims in ephedra-containing dietary supplements. *Am J Health Syst Pharm* 2000;57(10):963–9.
5. Kemper KJ, O'Connor KG. Pediatricians' recommendations for complementary and alternative medical (CAM) therapies. *Ambul Pediatr* 2004;4(6):482–7.
6. Sawyer MG, Gannoni AF, Toogood IR, et al. The use of alternative therapies by children with cancer. *Med J Aust* 1994;160(6):320–2.
7. Gupta D, Lis CG, Birdsall TC, et al. The use of dietary supplements in a community hospital comprehensive cancer center: implications for conventional cancer care. *Support Care Cancer* 2005;13(11):912–9.
8. McCune JS, Hatfield AJ, Blackburn AA, et al. Potential of chemotherapy-herb interactions in adult cancer patients. *Support Care Cancer* 2004;12(6):454–62.
9. Ioannidis JP, Hesketh PJ, Lau J. Contribution of dexamethasone to control of chemotherapy-induced nausea and vomiting: a meta-analysis of randomized evidence. *J Clin Oncol* 2000;18(19):3409–22.
10. Roscoe JA, Morrow GR, Hickok JT, et al. Nausea and vomiting remain a significant clinical problem: trends over time in controlling chemotherapy-induced nausea and vomiting in 1413 patients treated in community clinical practices. *J Pain Symptom Manage* 2000;20(2):113–21.
11. Block KI, Gyllenhaal C, Mead MN. Safety and efficacy of herbal sedatives in cancer care. *Integr Cancer Ther* 2004;3(2):128–48.
12. Kasper S, Anghelescu IG, Szegedi A, et al. Superior efficacy of St John's wort extract WS 5570 compared to placebo in patients with major depression: a randomized, double-blind, placebo-controlled, multi-center trial [ISRCTN77277298]. *BMC Med* 2006;4:14.
13. Mathijssen RH, Verweij J, de Bruijn P, et al. Effects of St. John's wort on irinotecan metabolism. *J Natl Cancer Inst* 2002;94(16):1247–9.

14. NIH. *Botanical Research Center Program.* [cited 2006 November 14]; Available from: http://dietary-supplements.info.nih.gov/Research/Dietary_Supplement_Research_Centers.aspx.
15. Franzblau SG, Cross C. Comparative in vitro antimicrobial activity of Chinese medicinal herbs. *J Ethnopharmacol* 1986;15(3):279–88.
16. Yang LQ, Singh M, Yap EH, et al. In vitro response of Blastocystis hominis against traditional Chinese medicine. *J Ethnopharmacol* 1996;55(1):35–42.
17. Zhang L, Yang L, Zheng X. A study of Helicobacterium pylori and prevention and treatment of chronic atrophic gastritis. *J Tradit Chin Med* 1997;17(1):3–9.
18. Song LC, Chen KZ, Zhu JY. [The effect of Coptis chinensis on lipid peroxidation and antioxidases activity in rats]. *Zhongguo Zhong Xi Yi Jie He Za Zhi* 1992;12(7):421–3, 390.
19. Wang GD, Zhang YM, Xiong XY. [Clinical and experimental study of burns treated locally with Chinese herbs]. *Zhong Xi Yi Jie He Za Zhi* 1991;11(12):727–9, 709.
20. Huang WM, Yan J, Xu J. [Clinical and experimental study on inhibitory effect of sanhuang mixture on platelet aggregation]. *Zhongguo Zhong Xi Yi Jie He Za Zhi* 1995;15(8):465–7.
21. Fang XP, Wang TZ, Zhang H, et al. [Quantitative determination of 5 alkaloids in plants of Coptis from China]. *Zhongguo Zhong Yao Za Zhi* 1989;14(2):33–5, 63.
22. Kobayashi Y, Yamashita Y, Fujii N, et al. Inhibitors of DNA topoisomerase I and II isolated from the Coptis rhizomes. *Planta Med* 1995;61(5):414–8.
23. Yamashita Y, Fujii N, Nakano H. Identification of novel topoisomerase I inhibitors. *Proc Amer Assoc Cancer Res* 1994;35:707.
24. Chi CW, Chang YF, Chao TW, et al. Flowcytometric analysis of the effect of berberine on the expression of glucocorticoid receptors in human hepatoma HepG2 cells. *Life Sci* 1994;54(26):2099–107.
25. Fukutake M, Yokota S, Kawamura H, et al. Inhibitory effect of Coptidis Rhizoma and Scutellariae Radix on azoxymethane-induced aberrant crypt foci formation in rat colon. *Biol Pharm Bull* 1998;21(8):814–7.
26. Qin CL, Liu JY, Cheng ZM. [Pharmacological studies on the effects of huanglian decoction on experimental gastric lesions in rats and antiemetic in pigeons]. *Zhongguo Zhong Yao Za Zhi* 1994;19(7):427–30, 448.
27. Gao XS. [Absorptive capacity of upper gastrointestinal tract with Chinese herbal medicine]. *Zhongguo Zhong Xi Yi Jie He Za Zhi* 1993;13(7):433–5, 390.
28. Ozaki Y, Suzuki H, Satake M. [Comparative studies on concentration of berberine in plasma after oral administration of coptidis rhizoma extract, its cultured cells extract, and combined use of these extracts and glycyrrhizae radix extract in rats]. *Yakugaku Zasshi* 1993;113(1):63–9.
29. Society AC. *Cancer Facts and Figures.* 2005 [cited 2006 November 14]; Available from: http://www.cancer.org/downloads/STT/CAFF2005f4PWSecured.pdf.
30. Society AC. *Estimated Cancer Deaths for Selected Cancer Sites.* 2006 [cited 2006 November 14].
31. Reis L, Hankey B, Miller B, *Cancer Statistics Review 1973–1988.* 1991, National Cancer Institute: Bethesda, Maryland.
32. Feld R, Rubinstein LV, Weisenberger TH. Sites of recurrence in resected stage I non-small-cell lung cancer: a guide for future studies. *J Clin Oncol* 1984;2(12):1352–8.
33. Shepherd FA, Dancey J, Ramlau R, et al. Prospective randomized trial of docetaxel versus best supportive care in patients with non-small-cell lung cancer previously treated with platinum-based chemotherapy. *J Clin Oncol* 2000;18(10):2095–103.
34. Vaporciyan A, Nesbitt J, Lee JS, et al., *Cancer of the Lung.* Cancer Medicine, ed. R. Bast, et al. 2002, Hamilton, Ontario: B.C. Decker Inc.
35. Lau BH, Ruckle HC, Botolazzo T, et al. Chinese medicinal herbs inhibit growth of murine renal cell carcinoma. *Cancer Biother* 1994;9(2):153–61.
36. Nagasawa H, Watanabe K, Yoshida M, et al. Effects of gold banded lily (Lilium auratum Lindl) or Chinese milk vetch (Astragalus sinicus L) on spontaneous mammary tumourigenesis in SHN mice. *Anticancer Res* 2001;21(4A):2323–8.

37. Sun Y, Hersh EM, Talpaz M, et al. Immune restoration and/or augmentation of local graft versus host reaction by traditional Chinese medicinal herbs. *Cancer* 1983;52(1):70–3.
38. Liu J. Analysis of the effects of TCM treatment according to syndrome differentiation in treating 310 cases of primary NSCLC. *Shanghai Tradit Chin Med J* 1985;10:3–6.
39. Liu J, Xu Z, Shi Z, et al. A prospective evaluation of TCM treatment according to Fuzheng Method in treating 122 cases of late stage primary NSCLC. *Acta Med Sinca* 1987;2(1):11–6.
40. Liu J, Shi Z, Guo Y, et al. Clinical study of TCM treatment according to "Nourishing Yin and Supplementing Qi" of late stage primary adenocarcinoma. *J Tradit Chin Med* 1995;36(3): 155–8.
41. Liu J, Shi Z, Li H, et al. Clinical observation on 271 cases of non-small lung cancer treated with Yifei Kangliu Yin (Jin Fu Kang). *Chin J Integr Tradit West Med* 2001;7(4):247–50.
42. Liu J, Shi Z, Xu Z, et al. Clinical observation on treatment of non-parvicellular carcinoma of the lung with jin fu kang oral liquid. *J Tradit Chin Med* 2000;20(2):96–100.
43. Liu J, Pan M, Li Y, et al. Clinical study of oral liquid Jin Fu Kang for the treatment of primary non-small cell lung cancer. *Tumor (Shanghai)* 2001;21(6):463–5.
44. McCulloch M, See C, Shu XJ, et al. Astragalus-based Chinese herbs and platinum-based chemotherapy for advanced non-small-cell lung cancer: meta-analysis of randomized trials. *J Clin Oncol* 2006;24(3):419–30.
45. Smigal C, Jemal A, Ward E, et al. Trends in breast cancer by race and ethnicity: update 2006. *CA Cancer J Clin* 2006;56(3):168–83..
46. Cui Y, Shu XO, Gao Y, et al. Use of complementary and alternative medicine by chinese women with breast cancer. *Breast Cancer Res Treat* 2004;85(3):263–70.
47. Bocca C, Gabriel L, Bozzo F, et al. A sesquiterpene lactone, costunolide, interacts with microtubule protein and inhibits the growth of MCF-7 cells. *Chem Biol Interact* 2004;147(1):79–86.
48. Campbell MJ, Hamilton B, Shoemaker M, et al. Antiproliferative activity of Chinese medicinal herbs on breast cancer cells in vitro. *Anticancer Res* 2002;22(6C):3843–52.
49. Jo EH, Hong HD, Ahn NC, et al. Modulations of the Bcl-2/Bax family were involved in the chemopreventive effects of licorice root (Glycyrrhiza uralensis Fisch) in MCF-7 human breast cancer cell. *J Agric Food Chem* 2004;52(6):1715–9.
50. Ohno N, Adachi Y, Suzuki I, et al. Antitumor activity of a beta-1,3-glucan obtained from liquid cultured mycelium of Grifola frondosa. *J Pharmacobiodyn* 1986;9(10):861–4.
51. Takeyama T, Suzuki I, Ohno N, et al. Host-mediated antitumor effect of grifolan NMF-5N, a polysaccharide obtained from Grifola frondosa. *J Pharmacobiodyn* 1987;10(11):644–51.
52. Suzuki I, Hashimoto K, Oikawa S, et al. Antitumor and immunomodulating activities of a beta-glucan obtained from liquid-cultured Grifola frondosa. *Chem Pharm Bull (Tokyo)* 1989;37(2):410–3.
53. Adachi K, Nanba H, Kuroda H. Potentiation of host-mediated antitumor activity in mice by beta-glucan obtained from Grifola frondosa (maitake). *Chem Pharm Bull (Tokyo)* 1987;35(1):262–70.
54. Suzuki I, Itani T, Ohno N, et al. Effect of a polysaccharide fraction from Grifola frondosa on immune response in mice. *J Pharmacobiodyn* 1985;8(3):217–26.
55. Kurashige S, Akuzawa Y, Endo F. Effects of Lentinus edodes, Grifola frondosa and Pleurotus ostreatus administration on cancer outbreak, and activities of macrophages and lymphocytes in mice treated with a carcinogen, N-butyl-N-butanolnitrosoamine. *Immunopharmacol Immunotoxicol* 1997;19(2):175–83.
56. Kodama N, Harada N, Nanba H. A polysaccharide, extract from Grifola frondosa, induces Th-I dominant response in BALB/c mice. *Jpn J Pharmacol* 2002;90(4):357–60.
57. Harada N, Kodama N, Nanba H. Relationship between dendritic cells and the D-fraction-induced Th-1 dominant response in BALB/c tumor-bearing mice. *Cancer Lett* 2003;192(2):181–7.
58. Nanba H. Maitake-D fracton: healing and preventive potential for cancer. *J Orthomol Med* 1997;12(1):43–9.
59. Kodama N, Komuta K, Nanba H. Can maitake MD-fraction aid cancer patients? *Altern Med Rev* 2002;7(3):236–9.

60. Lin H, She YH, Cassileth BR, et al. Maitake beta-glucan MD-fraction enhances bone marrow colony formation and reduces doxorubicin toxicity in vitro. *Int Immunopharmacol* 2004;4(1):91–9.
61. Bruix J, Barrera JM, Calvet X, et al. Prevalence of antibodies to hepatitis C virus in Spanish patients with hepatocellular carcinoma and hepatic cirrhosis. *Lancet* 1989;2(8670):1004–6.
62. Di Bisceglie A, Order S, Klein J. The role of chronic viral hepatitis in hepatocellular carcinoma in the United States. *Am J Gastroenterol* 1991;86:335–338.
63. Nishioka K, Watanabe J, Furuta S, et al. A high prevalence of antibody to the hepatitis C virus in patients with hepatocellular carcinoma in Japan. *Cancer* 1991;67(2):429–33.
64. McHutchison JG, Shad JA, Gordon SC, et al. Predicting response to initial therapy with interferon plus ribavirin in chronic hepatitis C using serum HCV RNA results during therapy. *J Viral Hepat* 2001;8(6):414–20.
65. Poynard T, Marcellin P, Lee SS, et al. Randomised trial of interferon alpha2b plus ribavirin for 48 weeks or for 24 weeks versus interferon alpha2b plus placebo for 48 weeks for treatment of chronic infection with hepatitis C virus. International Hepatitis Interventional Therapy Group (IHIT). *Lancet* 1998;352(9138):1426–32.
66. Scherin-Plough Kenilworth N. Rebetron. Package Insert. 2000.
67. van Rossum TG, Vulto AG, Hop WC, et al. Intravenous glycyrrhizin for the treatment of chronic hepatitis C: a double-blind, randomized, placebo-controlled phase I/II trial. *J Gastroenterol Hepatol* 1999;14(11):1093–9.
68. Inoue T, Jackson EK. Strong antiproliferative effects of baicalein in cultured rat hepatic stellate cells. *Eur J Pharmacol* 1999;378(1):129–35.
69. Li X, Wu XG. [Effects of ginseng on hepatocellular carcinoma in rats induced by diethylnitrosamine–a further study]. *J Tongji Med Univ* 1991;11(2):73–80.
70. Wu XG, Zhu DH. Influence of ginseng upon the development of liver cancer induced by diethylnitrosamine in rats. *J Tongji Med Univ* 1990;10(3):141–5, 133.
71. Yun YS, Lee YS, Jo SK, et al. Inhibition of autochthonous tumor by ethanol insoluble fraction from Panax ginseng as an immunomodulator. *Planta Med* 1993;59(6):521–4.
72. Konoshima T, Takasaki M, Ichiishi E, et al. Cancer chemopreventive activity of majonoside-R2 from Vietnamese ginseng, Panax vietnamensis. *Cancer Lett* 1999;147(1–2):11–6.
73. Miyamura M, Ono M, Kyotani S, et al. Effects of sho-saiko-to extract on fibrosis and regeneration of the liver in rats. *J Pharm Pharmacol* 1998;50(1):97–105.
74. Ono M, Miyamura M, Kyotani S, et al. Effects of Sho-saiko-to extract on liver fibrosis in relation to the changes in hydroxyproline and retinoid levels of the liver in rats. *J Pharm Pharmacol* 1999;51(9):1079–84.
75. Shimizu I, Ma YR, Mizobuchi Y, et al. Effects of Sho-saiko-to, a Japanese herbal medicine, on hepatic fibrosis in rats. *Hepatology* 1999;29(1):149–60.
76. Nagatsu Y, Inoue M, Ogihara Y. Modification of macrophage functions by Shosaikoto (kampo medicine) leads to enhancement of immune response. *Chem Pharm Bull (Tokyo)* 1989;37(6):1540–2.
77. Yamashiki M, Nishimura A, Nomoto M, et al. Herbal medicine 'Sho-saiko-to induces tumor necrosis factor-alpha and granulocyte colony-stimulating factor in vitro in peripheral blood mononuclear cells of patients with hepatocellular carcinoma. *J Gastroenterol Hepatol* 1996;11:137–42.
78. Sakaida I, Matsumura Y, Akiyama S, et al. Herbal medicine Sho-saiko-to (TJ-9) prevents liver fibrosis and enzyme-altered lesions in rat liver cirrhosis induced by a choline-deficient L-amino acid-defined diet. *J Hepatol* 1998;28(2):298–306.
79. Amagaya S, Hayakawa M, Ogihara Y, et al. Treatment of chronic liver injury in mice by oral administration of xiao-chai-hu-tang. *J Ethnopharmacol* 1989;25(2):181–7.
80. Tatsuta M, Iishi H, Baba M, et al. Inhibition by xiao-chai-hu-tang (TJ-9) of development of hepatic foci induced by N-nitrosomorpholine in Sprague-Dawley rats. *Jpn J Cancer Res* 1991;82(9):987–92.
81. Hirayama C, Okumura M, Tanikawa K, et al. A multicenter randomized controlled clinical trial of Shosaiko-to in chronic active hepatitis. *Gastroenterol Jpn* 1989;24(6):715–9.

82. Oka H, Yamamoto S, Kuroki T, et al. Prospective study of chemoprevention of hepatocellular carcinoma with Sho-saiko-to (TJ-9). *Cancer* 1995;76(5):743–9.
83. Sato A, Toyoshima M, Kondo A, et al. [Pneumonitis induced by the herbal medicine Sho-saiko-to in Japan]. *Nihon Kyobu Shikkan Gakkai Zasshi* 1997;35(4):391–5.
84. Ishak K, Baptista A, Bianchi L, et al. Histological grading and staging of chronic hepatitis. *J Hepatol* 1995;22(6):696–9.

Chapter 12
Acupuncture in Cancer Care at Dana-Farber Cancer Institute

An Integrative Medical Practice

Weidong Lu, Elizabeth Dean-Clower, Anne Doherty-Gilman and David S. Rosenthal

Contents

12.1	Overview and Background	182
12.2	Oncology Acupuncture, a New Medical Specialty?	185
12.3	Clinical Applications for Common Conditions in Cancer Care	187
12.4	Contraindications and Precautions in Acupuncture in Cancer Care	190
12.5	Acupuncture Use Inside a Cancer Center	191
	References	198

Abstract Acupuncture, an ancient form of medical treatment and philosophy originating in China over several thousand years ago, has gained increasing usage and acceptance in the United States over the past decade, including its use as adjunct treatment for cancer patients. Acupuncture is a major clinical service and focus of clinical research studies at the Leonard P. Zakim Center for Integrative Therapies at Dana-Farber Cancer Institute, in Boston, Massachusetts. The Zakim Center provides acupuncture for patients with cancer and cancer survivors for symptom management or treatment-related side effects, including chemotherapy-induced nausea/vomiting, cancer pain, insomnia, fatigue, anxiety, and/or a sense of well-being, based on the patient's condition and evidence of safety and efficacy. Communication with allopathic clinicians and documentation in the medical record are standard procedures in the Zakim Center which are crucial to the acupuncturist and the oncology care team members benefit from each other's contributions to the patient's overall cancer care. The successful integration of acupuncture at Dana-Farber, a premier academic

---

D. Rosenthal
Director, Harvard University Health Service, Co-Director, Zakim Center for Integrative Therapies, Dana-Farber Cancer Institute, Professor of Medicine, Harvard Medical School, Henry K. Oliver Professor of Hygiene, Harvard University, 75 Mount Auburn St., Cambridge, MA 02138, e-mail: drose@uhs.harvard.edu

medical and research facility, underscores the need for oncology acupuncture protocols and for more acupuncturists with specialized clinical experience working with cancer patients. For this reason, oncology acupuncture is proposed as a new subspecialty in which acupuncturists possess clinical knowledge and skills in both acupuncture and oncology in order to optimize safety and efficacy, thereby providing a truly integrative approach for the cancer patient population.

Keywords: Acupuncture · research · oncology acupuncture; electroacupuncture · cancer symptom management · treatment side effects · non-pharmaceutical intervention.

12.1 Overview and Background

Acupuncture is a major clinical service in the Leonard P. Zakim Center for Integrative Therapies (ZCIT) at the Dana-Farber Cancer Institute (DFCI), Boston, Massachusetts. The Center provides acupuncture for patients with cancer and cancer survivors, while conducting clinical trials in acupuncture as a main focus of research. But how did providing this on-site service at an academic research facility in the Harvard Medical arena come about?

Many U.S. clinicians have limited familiarity with acupuncture. This ancient form of medical treatment and philosophy originating in China over several thousand years ago is based on a very different theoretical framework than allopathic Western medicine. Over the past decade, acupuncture has gained increasing usage and acceptance in the United States as a valid medical intervention. Based on a consensus conference in 1997, the National Institutes of Health has defined acupuncture as "a family of procedures involving stimulation of anatomic locations on the skin by a variety of techniques. The most studied mechanism of stimulation of acupuncture points uses penetration of the skin by thin, solid, metallic needles, which are manipulated manually or by electrical stimulation [1]." While the National Institute of Health (NIH) definition itself seems reductionistic of this more complex medical practice, it reflected an important milestone in its recognition that acupuncture warranted further study and review using an evidenced-based approach.

12.1.1 Acupuncture at DFCI

When the Zakim Center first opened in November 2000, acupuncture was chosen as one of the first clinical interventions at the Center. This choice was made not only because patients were requesting it, but also because of its safety and reported efficacy. While known for its biomedical research and teaching hospitals, Boston also benefits from a strong professional community of acupuncturists, particularly given the local expertise of faculty of the New England School of Acupuncture in Watertown, Massachusetts, one of the oldest acupuncture schools in the United States. Also, although acupuncture has been a less frequently used complementary and alternative medical (CAM) therapy by the general population, with more clinical and basic scientific evidence available to assure that it would be clinically helpful and well-received by both patients and their physicians, acupuncture was introduced at DFCI and an acupuncture policy was introduced (see Chapter 7, Table 1). Often Chinese herbal medicine (CHM) is used in combination with acupuncture as an integral part of Traditional Chinese Medicine (TCM) treatment, but because DFCI oncologists expressed concern about the safe use of Chinese herbs with their patients' care plans due to the potential drug–herb interactions and the quality and consistency of such products, we decided to offer acupuncture without the use of CHM. Acupuncture in conventional cancer care was relatively new and innovative in the United States, and as will be discussed, there were many challenges integrating this service into our comprehensive cancer center.

During the 2000–2006, over 6000 acupuncture treatments have been delivered at DFCI for various clinical symptoms. Acupuncture is a reasonable option for cancer patients given the nature of their symptoms and side effects from conventional therapies, such as chemotherapy-induced nausea/vomiting, cancer pain, insomnia, fatigue and anxiety. Acupuncture is used at all stages of cancer: patients who are newly diagnosed and beginning to make treatment decisions; patients who are in the midst of chemotherapy or radiation therapy and experiencing side effects; patients who have completed cancer treatment and are in a transition period rehabilitating back to their normal life; and patients who have been off treatment for years, but want to enhance their immune system, quality of life, or general sense of well-being.

As mentioned, Chinese medicine has a very different theoretical framework than conventional medicine. For example, a cancer patient with depression is often described as "Liver Qi Stagnation" in Chinese medicine; a patient undergoing chemotherapy with neutropenia is seen as "Qi and Blood Deficiency." In theory, two patients with the same cancer diagnosis and stage would not be treated the same way with respect to acupuncture. Major differences also exist in the treatment strategies and in the detailed descriptions of the acupuncture points among acupuncturists with different styles. Many acupuncturists are not educated about the clinical implication and consequences of oncologic treatment, such as a patient undergoing chemotherapy developing febrile neutropenia. These discordances pose potential risks to patient safety and clinical services. It may seem counterintuitive to perform an invasive procedure, albeit minimally so, involving any form of needles, on patients who may be susceptible to infection or are on anticoagulation. Yet when acupuncture is properly carried out with certain safeguards in place e.g., single use, sterilized needles, thorough knowledge of anatomy and blood labs results, modification of technique if anticoagulation therapy is used, and written permission of the primary oncologist (see Chapter 7, Fig. 1)], acupuncture is both safe and potentially beneficial. It is crucial that both the acupuncturist and the oncology care team understand each other in order to establish effective communication and understanding so the patients can truly benefit from an integrative approach.

12.1.2 Documentation

The documentation of acupuncture procedures is important and should be concise, clear and interpretable. The practitioner should always be aware that his or her documentation is part of the medical record and will be reviewed and interpreted by other members of the patient care team. In order to achieve such integration, the acupuncturist needs to minimize the use of special terms unique to Chinese medicine. Instead, general descriptive terms should be used to document the patient symptoms, conditions and treatment approaches. Because acupuncture is used in cancer patients mostly as supportive care and symptom management, we have found that the diagnostic terms that are unique to Chinese medicine are usually not necessary. The important message is if any TCM terms to be used, it should always give a general description, followed by the specific terms, so the other members of the team understand the meaning and confusion is avoided. Therefore, an acupuncturist assessing a patient's condition should also possess adequate clinical knowledge and understanding of western medicine. Commonly used medical terms should be used to clearly and accurately describe the patient's condition and history.

TCM terms written without description should generally be avoided if possible such as "Liver Yang Rising," or "Kidney Qi Deficiency." For example, if the patient is felt to have "Kidney Qi Deficiency," and it must be documented the term can be written as "Kidney Qi Deficiency, a TCM term that generally describes a patient with reduced vital energies that pertain to the endocrine and reproductive systems," or "Liver Yang Rising, a TCM term that describes a patient with physical symptoms and signs such as headaches, red complexion, mouth sores, and emotional distress like agitation or restlessness." TCM terms regarding anatomy such as "Liver," "Spleen" and so on should be put in quotations to avoid misunderstandings regarding anatomy by other health care professionals reading the medical record note.

For acupuncturists who are interested in documenting the specific "pattern diagnosis" from the Chinese medicine perspective, it is recommended to describe in detail the key symptoms that encompass that particular term. For example, rather than writing "this patient has Qi and Blood Deficiency," it is better to describe the condition as "the patient demonstrates fatigue, shortness of breath, aversion to cold, along with anemia."

Another important reason to use a descriptive style of documentation is to monitor the effects of treatments provided by different members of the medical team. However, some unique and well-accepted TCM terms should be kept in medical records. For example, the "De Qi" (a slightly achy sensation during needling that relates to treatment effects) should be noted.

When assessing the patient's condition and the treatment plan, it is important to document a clear recommendation of the proposed treatment which should include the recommended treatment, the frequency, and the expected treatment results.

Explaining TCM terminology is an effective strategy that helps to overcome the language barrier between TCM and conventional medicine clinicians. However, such a strategy does not preclude the discussions of the individual concepts in the two medical traditions amongst the oncology care team members. In fact, such discussions and exchanges should be encouraged, as they may enhance safety and efficacy, are academically interesting, and may generate potential research questions.

12.1.3 Developing Standardized Acupuncture Protocols

In the traditional practice of Chinese medicine, individualization of treatment is considered a norm, and a standardized approach is considered to be overly rigid and less effective. However, such a nation is yet to be supported by data and raises concerns regarding reproducibility and in conducting evidence-based research. Acupuncture in an oncology practice focuses on symptom management and enhancement of QOL. The clinical conditions of oncology patients are highly variable, especially during chemotherapy. Therefore, a standardized protocol of acupuncture for commonly seen symptoms is urgently needed. This approach would minimize practice variability and improve patient safety. The treatment protocol requires support from previous clinical studies, data analysis and consensus of experienced oncology acupuncturists. Currently, standardized protocols are yet to be established.

12.2 Oncology Acupuncture, a New Medical Specialty?

Oncology acupuncture could become a new subspecialty in which clinicians possess clinical knowledge and skills in both acupuncture and oncology. An oncology acupuncturist uses acupuncture as a non-pharmaceutical intervention to treat physical and emotional symptoms of cancer patients and survivors and to minimize the side effects of various cancer therapies and improve the quality of life. An oncology acupuncturist is part of the pain and symptom management team in a cancer program and works closely with other specialists in medical and radiation oncology, psychosocial oncologists and nursing specialists.

12.2.1 Requirements and Challenges for an Oncology Acupuncturist

In order to fulfil the clinical tasks as an oncology acupuncturist, we propose the following necessary requirements:

- An acupuncture license
- A general medical training background
- Hospital system experience, good communication skills, and cultural competence
- Experience treating oncology patients

First, the oncology acupuncturist should have a comprehensive training in acupuncture and in Chinese medicine, usually from an accredited acupuncture school, licensed by a state authority. This training equips the clinician with a broad knowledge in needling techniques, acupuncture point selection, treatment options and strategies of acupuncture. However, this curriculum is not sufficient to ensure that the clinician is capable of safely treating oncology patients as most training programs currently available in U.S. acupuncture schools do not address the specific clinical needs of cancer patients.

The second recommendation is that the clinician needs to have training in general medicine in order to recognize and interpret medical conditions and perform an oncology acupuncture evaluation. Clinical knowledge in cancer biology, diagnoses, staging, treatments and prognosis is important. Although the acupuncturist is not required to manage medical emergencies, it is critical for the practitioner to recognize potential risks and possible oncologic emergencies while administering acupuncture treatment. Clinical skills such as understanding and interpreting basic laboratory values, biological cancer markers and their clinical significance are essential in working with a cancer population. The practitioner should be able to understand reports from the radiology imaging department, such as magnetic resonance imaging (MRI), computed tomography scans and ultrasound exams, in order to monitor the effect of interventions and the appropriateness of various acupuncture strategies.

The third requirement is that an oncology acupuncturist needs to have knowledge and working experience in a hospital setting with skills to effectively communicate with other members of a multidisciplinary medical team. In addition, for a clinician with an international background, overcoming cultural barriers may be necessary. Because various schools of thought currently exist in the acupuncture profession, it is imperative for an acupuncturist to communicate the treatment rationale and clinical decision-making process with other acupuncture team members.

The fourth requirement is that the practitioner needs to have experience working with cancer patients. Although almost every acupuncturist has treated a few patients with cancer in their community practice, it requires frequent and intensive clinical encounters with cancer patients to develop a competency in this field.

Unfortunately, at this time, there are few practitioners who have met all of these criteria in a systematic way. Acupuncturists who are currently working with cancer patients may be mostly self-trained or self-claimed. The quality of care is thus of concern. Table 2 in Chapter 7 is DFCI's current approach to credentialing acupuncturists in the ambulatory or patient setting.

12.2.2 Potential Sources of Oncology Acupuncturists

Licensed acupuncturists, physician acupuncturists, oncology nurses and other trained health care providers could potentially be oncology acupuncturists with proper training.

As most acupuncturists currently trained in acupuncture schools in the United States focus on the classical TCM diagnosis and treatment approaches, they may not be familiar with conventional ambulatory practice of medicine. They may lack knowledge and experience in interpreting medical data, as well as handling the emergencies encountered in the oncology practice. Nevertheless acupuncturists have unique skills to contribute to the multidisciplinary team if they receive additional clinical oncologic training.

Some graduates from traditional Chinese medical schools in China have received training in both classical TCM and western medicine. They practice as licensed acupuncturists in the United States and may require minimal additional training before being hired as oncology acupuncturists, such as improving communication skills.

At DFCI, we started our acupuncture program with two acupuncturists who used different styles of acupuncture, Chinese and Japanese. We found it difficult to transfer patient care between acupuncturists because they were using different techniques. We learned that the acupuncture team should be comprised of acupuncturists who use the same style of acupuncture as much as possible. We now have four acupuncturists on staff, all of whom were trained in China. They each hold a medical degree from Chinese medical schools in Traditional Chinese Medicine, have clinical experience working in a hospital environment, have more than 10 years of clinical experience in TCM and hold an acupuncture license from the Board of Registration in Medicine in the Commonwealth of Massachusetts. As faculty members of the New England School of Acupuncture in Watertown, Massachusetts, they all teach at least one acupuncture course and/or supervise a student acupuncture clinic. Because they have a similar training background in acupuncture, they are able to deliver a consistent treatment to patients, using the same acupuncture techniques. This also helps for clinical trials, solving a significant issue of variability in the acupuncture profession involved in clinical research.

Physician acupuncturists trained in U.S. hospitals and licensed to practice medicine in United States have had some level of acupuncture training. Although these physicians have knowledge to deal with medical issues, patient assessment and treatments of cancer patients, most of their acupuncture training is obtained through weekend courses or distance learning and may not be adequate to deal with oncology acupuncture issues. Nevertheless, this shortcoming could be countered by their clinical experience in acupuncture practice.

In summary, there is currently a gap between the clinical needs and the availability of qualified and competent oncology acupuncturists. There are few readily available oncology acupuncturists currently in the United States. Establishing a training program for currently practicing acupuncturists is urgently needed. A program at Memorial Sloan-Kettering Cancer Center, entitled "Integrating Acupuncture into Mainstream Cancer Treatment Centers," is one example of such a program.

12.3 Clinical Applications for Common Conditions in Cancer Care

Acupuncture is being practiced more and more for patients with cancer at different times during the continuum of their cancer treatment. It is important for patients with cancer to understand that acupuncture is used as supportive therapy to minimize the cancer treatment's side effects and improve their quality of life. Current medical evidence does not support any claim that acupuncture should be used as an "alternative" to conventional cancer therapy.

The use of acupuncture in oncology care is increasing, and with more evidence-based research being published, clinical efficacy data are now available for some clinical cancer-related problems, but is still limited.

12.3.1 Acupuncture for Chemotherapy-Induced Nausea/Vomiting

Acupuncture has been studied for chemotherapy-induced nausea and vomiting since early 1990s. Several large randomized clinical trials indicate that acupuncture is an effective therapy for reducing the severity and frequency of these side effects. In 1997, the NIH consensus statement on acupuncture declared: "There is clear evidence that needle acupuncture is efficacious for adult postoperative and chemotherapy nausea and vomiting and probably for the nausea of pregnancy" [1].

A randomized controlled trial led by Shen in 2000 [2] further confirmed acupuncture's antiemetic effect for patients receiving chemotherapy, with a significant reduction of mean emesis episodes (5 versus 15; $P < .001$) compared with pharmacotherapy alone.

Two important clinical notes from the trial were generated:

1. Electroacupuncture yielded a more effective response than conventional acupuncture.
2. The most effective acupuncture point was PC-6.

12.3.2 Acupuncture for Radiotherapy-Induced Xerostomia

Several pilot clinical studies suggest that acupuncture may improve xerostomia, the dry mouth condition caused by radiation therapy for patients with head and neck cancer [3]. Dr. Peter Johnstone and his colleagues used acupuncture for patients with pilocarpine-resistant xerostomia after radiotherapy for head and neck cancer. He found a 70% response rate with an increase of 10% or more from the baseline Xerostomia Inventory [4,5].

The technique for treating xerostomia includes placing acupuncture needles along the anatomical distribution of major salivary glands, the parotid gland, submandibular gland and sublingual gland. The ear point named San Jiao (Triple Warmer) is a common point associated with clinical response. Electroacupuncture can enhance the beneficial results.

A similar clinical benefit at DFCI has also been noted. In some cases, it was found that patients could still respond to the acupuncture for this condition several years after the completion of radiotherapy.

12.3.3 Acupuncture for Post-Chemotherapy-Related Fatigue

Vickers reported that acupuncture was helpful in managing persistent fatigue among cancer patients who had previously completed cytotoxic chemotherapy. The mean improvement from baseline fatigue score was 31.3% (95% CI: 20.6–41.5%) [6].

Patients who have completed their chemotherapy treatment and still experience persistent fatigue several months later may be encouraged to use acupuncture. Clinically, acupuncture needling should be gentle but consistent. Acupuncture points of selection are ST36, SP6, Yintang, GV20 and GV24. Noticeable improvement is expected even at the end of one course. At the DFCI acupuncture clinic, we find that for patients who are undergoing chemotherapy and/or radiotherapy and who are complaining of severe fatigue, a course of 6–8 weekly acupuncture sessions can greatly improve their energy level.

12.3.4 Acupuncture for Chemotherapy-Related Neuropathy

Chemotherapy-induced peripheral neuropathy is a common side effect of cancer therapy. Similar symptoms are seen among patients with diabetes and other drug-induced neuropathic pain. Wong and Sagar reported a small study of five patients who had a partial response to acupuncture treatment that could not be easily explained by the known neurophysiologic mechanisms of acupuncture [7]. Although higher levels of evidence are still lacking in this area, using acupuncture and/or electrostimulation for diabetes neuropathy has been reported. The findings suggest that acupuncture may be a safe and effective therapy for the long-term management of painful diabetic neuropathy. At DFCI, we have observed a reduction of neuropathic pain and improvement of abnormal sensations in the extremities in some patients with chemotherapy related neuropathy. We have found that it is best to use acupuncture at the earliest signs and symptoms of neuropathy.

12.3.5 Acupuncture for Cancer Pain

In a randomized, placebo controlled clinical trial, Alimi et al. [8] reported a 36% reduction of pain from baseline at 2 months using ear acupuncture among patients with chronic peripheral or central neuropathic pain arising after treatment of a cancer.

In our DFCI clinic, our experience is that patients report that acupuncture for cancer pain is helpful, especially, among patients who have completed cancer treatments. Using acupuncture as an adjunct therapy for patients who require narcotic support for pain may provide additive clinical benefits.

12.3.6 Acupuncture for Insomnia and Anxiety

Several non-cancer-related clinical trials suggest that acupuncture is an effective method to reduce the anxiety level of preoperative patients [9, 10]. In a group of women with chronic neck and shoulder pain, a study found a significant improvement in their sleep pattern, anxiety level and quality of life in addition to the improvement of pain level [11]. These improvements remained significant 6 months after the completion of the study. Acupuncture is also reported to help improve the sleep quality in patients with insomnia and anxiety [12].

In the DFCI clinic, we have noticed that a reduction of anxiety level is an early indication of a "responder" toward acupuncture treatment. The majority of cancer patients treated at DFCI reported a satisfactory relaxation immediately after just one acupuncture session.

Clinically, acupuncture for this group of patients should be gentle and the number of the points selected limited. Use of electroacupuncture should be avoided for some patients but may be effective once the patient feels more comfortable with the procedure.

12.3.7 Acupuncture for Other Clinical Issues

Cancer treatment induced early menopause symptoms; radiotherapy-induced trismus (lock jaw); chemotherapy-induced leukopenia, chemotherapy-induced diarrhea; postoperative pain and end of life care are all areas when acupuncture may be of help. Most cancer patients also have non-cancer-related symptoms that greatly affect their quality of life during the cancer treatment, such as back pain, headaches and myalgia. These can also be addressed by acupuncture.

12.4 Contraindications and Precautions in Acupuncture in Cancer Care

12.4.1 Neutropenia

Neutropenia is the most common side effect of chemotherapy. Some preliminary studies suggest that acupuncture might be beneficial for patients with chemotherapy-induced neutropenia. However, results indicate that this benefit is mild to moderate, generally in patients with grade 1 to grade 2 neutropenia ($1000–2000/mm^3$). When a patient's absolute neutrophil count (ANC) drops to $500/mm^3$, acupuncture treatment should be withheld until the ANC value rises above $500/mm^3$. Closely monitoring the ANC level during chemotherapy is a critical component to protect the patient's safety.

When treating a patient undergoing chemotherapy, the acupuncturist should be aware of the nature of the chemotherapy, for example, the type of myelosuppressive agent used and the chemotherapy cycles, to predict the nadir. If there has been a previous episode of febrile neutropenia, acupuncture should be avoided during the expected nadir.

12.4.2 Thrombocytopenia

Thrombocytopenia, a platelet count of less than $140,000/mm^3$, may occur after high doses of chemotherapy. Acupuncture is not considered a contraindication for mild thrombocytopenia, that is, grade 1 or grade 2, $100,000-140,000/mm^3$. However, if the patient has moderate, thrombocytopenia (50–100,000), then deep needle insertion should be avoided. If the platelet count is below $25,000/mm^3$, acupuncture should be delayed until the patient's platelets count rises above $25,000/mm^3$.

12.4.3 Anticoagulants

Cancer is a risk factor for venous thromboembolism. Anticoagulant use in these cases is monitored by the International Normalization Ratio (INR) and generally range between 2.0 and 3.0.

In our experience, acupuncture does not increase the chance of bleeding in this population. However, the practitioner should be aware of the risk of bleeding and avoid deep needling and strong stimulation. Compressing needling holes after withdrawing needles is recommended.

12.4.4 Metastatic Sites

The most common metastatic sites of cancer are lungs, liver, brain and bones. When encountering a patient with a known history of cancer complaining of bone pain, the practitioner should refer the patient back to the oncologist to exclude the possibility of cancer metastasis before any acupuncture treatment is given. Inserting acupuncture needles into a metastatic site should be absolutely avoided as the clinical consequences are still unknown. Careful history taking, physical exam and appropriate imaging tests (X-ray, MRI, and CT scan) would help to clarify the cause of the pain.

12.5 Acupuncture Use Inside a Cancer Center

12.5.1 Daily Clinical Pathways of Acupuncture Care

Practicing acupuncture in a cancer canter is very different than practicing acupuncture in a community setting. Facing different patient populations, patients with co-morbid medical conditions and interactions with professional staff are just a few of the challenges.

12.5.2 Pre-Clinical Time Preparations

12.5.2.1 Materials and Set Ups

Room

A regular ambulatory clinic exam room can be converted into an acupuncture treatment room with minor changes. A regular exam table can be used as the treatment table; however, it may not be as comfortable as a massage table with strong supportive legs, which provides a firm and soft surface.

The treatment room should provide an appropriately warm, quiet, environment, equipped with necessary emergency support and wall outlets. The room needs to be equipped with regular medical equipment, such as oxygen wall outlets, emergency buttons, a blood pressure wall unit, and so on. The room temperature should generally be set at 72–75°F. A slightly warmer room temperature is important, because patients during treatment often experience a drop in body temperature that may be uncomfortable. The lighting should be soft on the dim side, but adequate enough to perform the procedure. Direct light into the eyes should be avoided. Ideally, the treatment room should be in a quiet, less trafficked area of the clinic floor in order to avoid unnecessary disturbances. A dressing mirror is recommended for the patients who need to dress up after finishing the treatment, particularly cancer patients who might have alopecia. The treatment room should have decorative amenities with gentle and relaxing music available to distinguish it from a medical exam room.

Many acupuncture treatments can be performed in open ambulatory areas, such as infusion rooms. However, a full-body treatment is not appropriate for those settings.

Needles

Food and Drug Administration (FDA)-approved acupuncture needles with various sizes and length are recommended. Commonly used needle sizes are 1 inch/36 gauge and 1.5 inch/36 or 32 gauges in Chinese style needles. Japanese styled acupuncture needles like brand Seirin® needles No. 1 and No. 2. are also used. Other size needles can be used depending on the patient size and the locations of the site to be needled.

Moxibustion

Use of moxibustion in a hospital setting is not recommended (burning a moxa stick would produce a strong smoke-like odor) because it presents a fire hazard in an oxygen-rich environment, could easily burn the patient's skin and could irritate patients who are particularly sensitive to smells, a common occurrence when cancer patients are undergoing treatment.

Cupping

Cupping for patients undergoing active chemotherapy and radiotherapy is not recommended. Caution should be used with the cupping technique as many cancer patients bruise easily. In our practice, when patients have completed their active chemotherapy and/or radiotherapy and blood counts are back to normal, cupping can be considered.

Infrared Heat Lamp

There are two types of heat lamps used alongside acupuncture. One is a fast-heated, infrared heat lamp and the other is the TDP infrared heat lap. Each has its pros and cons. The purpose of the heat lamp is to replace moxibustion as a source of heat and also to provide a comforting environment, warming the extremities of the patient during the resting session. In addition, heat lamps promote local blood circulation, which can enhance the effects of the acupuncture treatment. Some studies suggest the acupuncture clinical outcome relates to the skin temperature of the patient during the treatment. Maintaining a warm skin temperature is an important part of the acupuncture treatment [13,4].

12.5.2.2 Electroacupuncture Device

In addition to the basic acupuncture needles, one electrical acupuncture stimulator is recommended. FDA registered units should be used, preferably those with a digital reading, which precisely control the treatment frequency.

12.5.2.3 Other Materials

A timer and handheld wireless chiming device/doorbell are essential during the acupuncture, so that patients are able to communicate with the acupuncturist directly during the resting session. Wireless devices serve to minimize the patient's restlessness and anxicty, particularly during the first few treatments.

12.5.3 Record Review Prior To Treatment

Prior to the clinic visit, the acupuncturist needs to set up the required treatment equipment and ensure the appropriate environment. The patient's medical record should then be reviewed from either the paper or the electronic medical records system, including the laboratory studies (see Chapter 7, Fig. 2). The vital signs of the patients should be performed before each visit and include the pulse, the temperature, blood pressure, respiratory rate, weight and body mass index. Next, review the previous notes of the last acupuncture visit if applicable. Attention should be given to all clinical notes that occurred between last visit and today's visit, by all members of the health care team including any emergency room visits and regular checkups.

Next, review the latest laboratory values. Special attention should be given to the hematology results including complete blood counts (CBC), that is, WBC, RBC, Hgb, HCT and PLT with the WBC differential as well. Attention should be given especially to the ANC. For patients currently receiving chemotherapy, the flow sheet of drugs should be reviewed.

12.5.4 New Patients

During the first visit, enough time should be given to review their complete medical history and their medications. To obtain complete understanding of the patient's current medical condition, from the oncology perspective, the acupuncturist should understand the diagnosis, oncology diagnosis, the tumor stages and the site of the tumor locations. The acupuncturist should assure the patient's oncologist has confirmed that the patient is eligible for treatment (see Chapter 7, Fig. 1). At DFCI, this form is emailed to the patient's oncology care team by our practice coordinator before the visit. A reply from the primary oncologist must be received in order for the treatment to commence.

A consent form should be signed before the acupuncture procedure and the procedure and the potential side effects should be discussed, such as bleeding, local pain and slight bruising around needle sides.

The acupuncturist should become aware of the stage of the tumor, whether there are metastases, and the treatment plan including surgery, chemotherapy and/or radiation therapy. The laboratory values should always be reviewed, for example, the CBC, the BUN, creatinine and the liver function tests. Attention should be given to any coagulation values, especially the INR.

Specific attention should be given to nutrition status, fever, gastrointestinal symptoms, physical activity, symptoms of fatigue, muscle weakness, shortness of breath, headache and insomnia. A pain assessment should be done using a standardized method. All medications should be reviewed and special attention should be given to whether the medications are used for symptom management. These medications could greatly influence the complaints of the patients and their reactions toward acupuncture treatments. Referrals to the other members of the oncology care team should be made as needed.

12.5.5 History Taking

The history should include the following areas: confirmation of at least two patient identifiers, for example, hospital number and date of birth, the diagnosis, the stage of the cancer and the current therapy. The history of the present illness will generally be a narrative description of the symptoms associated with the treatment. Visual analog scales are recommended to describe the degree or level of the condition to be recorded.

Past medical history, family medical history and social history should be obtained and reviewed. Specific attention should be given to the patient's occupation, marriage status, lifestyle, whether the patient is taking any specific vitamins, food supplements and/or herbs.

A brief physical exam should also be preformed for new patients, although for an acupuncture treatment, comprehensive physical exams are not necessary. The general appearance of the patient and the specific area to be needled needs to be documented and the findings need to be described from a TCM perspective, describing the tongue and the pulse specifically.

12.5.5.1 Assessment

This section should include the patient's prior experience with acupuncture and the patient's expectations regarding acupuncture treatment. The acupuncturist should give his/her own assessment and treatment plan, the number of treatments and the frequency of the treatment, and possible expectations of the treatment. A clear defined treatment goal should be given, with reference to short- and long-term goals when applicable.

The Karnofsky Performance Status (KPS) Scale is a very useful tool in assessing the patient. In general, a patient with a Karnofsky scale above 50% is suitable for acupuncture in an ambulatory setting. At that level, the patient may not able to work but is able to live at home and care for most personal needs. For patients with KPS score below 40%, acupuncture may not be appropriate for an ambulatory clinic. Patients below 40% are unable to care for self, require the equivalent of institutional or hospital care. The patient is disabled and requires special care and assistance. At 30% level, the patient is severely disabled, and hospital admission may be indicated. The ECOG Performance Status is another useful indicator. A patient with an ECOG grade 3 or above is eligible to receive acupuncture treatment in an ambulatory setting. At grade 3 of ECOG, performance status indicates the patient is capable of limited self-care, confined to a bed or chair more than 50% of their waking hours. Grade 4 indicates complete disability and completely confined to bed or chair, therefore unsuitable for acupuncture treatment in an ambulatory setting.

Acupuncture usually requires a course of treatment, that is, six or more continuous, weekly or semi-weekly treatments. It is important that the patient be able to travel to the clinic or that it is done in the hospital so as not to compromise the outcome of the treatment. Reasons that may deter patients from receiving acupuncture treatments are commute, depression, motivation as well as their medical conditions. For this group of patients, acupuncture can be given at an in-patient unit or home for end of life care.

12.5.5.2 Procedures

The last section of the acupuncture note should describe the acupuncture treatment preformed that day and include the following:

- Identification of the patient.
- The reason for the visit to the acupuncturist, that is, the symptoms such as pain, nausea, fatigue.
- Changes since last visit.
- Acupuncture procedure: detailed description of the patient's position on the massage table and the skin preparation, the acupuncture needles used including size and length of insertion and name of the acupuncture point. The internationally accepted names of the acupuncture points should be used. Comments should indicate whether there was manipulation of the needles and whether the sensation "De Qi" was experienced. The use of infrared heat lamp and/or electroacupuncture should also be described. The number of needles inserted, the duration of needle retaining time, and the number of needles removed at end of each session should be documented.
- Finally, the patient's relaxation and their reaction should be documented as well. All the treatment procedures and patient responses should be timely noted in the medical records.

In summary, it is important for acupuncturists to actively explain and describe how an acupuncture procedure is performed and provide a detailed description of the procedure, the goals of the therapy, as well as the intent of the treatment for a particular patient and a specific medical condition being treated.

12.5.6 Clinical Referral Paths of Acupuncture Care

12.5.6.1 Integrative Medical Consultation

Usually conducted by a senior oncologist, integrative medical consultations serve a central piece in an integrative medicine program. Patients are seeking the guidance and recommendations from an oncologist perspective. In addition, the consultation gives the oncologist a first hand clinical impression on the appropriateness of the medical conditions of the patients going to a specific integrative therapy. At DFCI, three physicians including the medical director have offered integrative medicine consults to patients and have referred appropriate patients to acupuncture treatments. Acupuncturists often refer patients for an integrative medical consultation if the patient has more clinical questions that may not relate to acupuncture but other complementary or alternative therapies that are best addressed by a physician.

12.5.6.2 Medical Oncologists

At DFCI, acupuncturists are part of the multi-disciplinary clinical team. It is crucial to assure close communication in collaboration with patient issues. Because acupuncture is a relatively new modality to many health care providers, and staff appropriately have various questions and concerns regarding particular patients and the appropriateness of acupuncture. The members of a medical team should meet with the acupuncturists and have regular meetings and discussions on the use and benefit of acupuncture therapy in cancer patients. Acupuncturists need to skilfully answer and explain the potential risks and the benefits so that the members of the medical team will feel comfortable with the treatment strategy and plan. The clinical operations should be set up so that practice coordinators contact the oncologists to confirm the patient's eligibility before the patient sees the acupuncturists. Acupuncturists should seek medical approval for each patient, from the treating oncologist using predefined eligibility criteria.

It is important for the acupuncturist to communicate regularly with the treating oncologist, discussing the responses or lack there of from the acupuncture. Many acupuncturists may not have adequate medical background and knowledge, especially in the oncology field, to accurately assess a cancer patient's clinical situation and prognosis. Therefore, receiving the support and assessment from the oncologist will greatly facilitate the treatment results and planning.

The medical oncologist, the care team leader, who is ultimately responsible for the outcome of the patient, is encouraged to ensure the patient's safety by fully understanding the role of acupuncture in the medical team.

12.5.6.3 Oncology Nurse Practitioners

An oncologist nurse practitioner plays a significant role in an oncology team. The oncologist nurse practitioner works closely with the oncologist and evaluates the progression of the disease and administers the chemotherapy and/or radiation therapy. We have found them to be accessible and willing to work with acupuncturists in managing the side effects of cancer therapies.

12.5.6.4 Nutritionists

Nutritionists are valuable members of the multidisciplinary team. They often respond to questions of dietary supplements and other complementary modalities. Acupuncturists and nutritionists often work together to manage issues like weight, nausea and gastro intestinal (GI) symptoms.

12.5.6.5 Physical Therapists

Cancer patients who require physical therapy generally have had surgical procedures. Physical therapists often closely work with acupuncturists in managing muscular injuries, postoperative recovery and chronic pain conditions. They usually have a good understanding of acupuncture as both disciplines involve working with structural and physical medicine, muscles and tendons.

12.5.6.6 Pain and Palliative Care Management

Acupuncturists should be a part of a pain and palliative care specialty clinical team in a cancer hospital because many of the therapeutic goals of acupuncture are within the scope of pain management. Moreover, acupuncture as a non-pharmaceutical intervention is a reasonable complementary to the drug-oriented pain management. At DFCI, the acupuncture service was initially housed in the Pain and Symptom Management Program, under the physician Director of Pain and Symptom Management.

12.5.6.7 Other CAM Practitioners

In larger cancer centers, in addition to acupuncture, there may be other CAM practitioners, such as massage therapists, music therapists and reiki masters. Two-way referrals frequently occur and should be encouraged among this group of therapists. As an acupuncturist, it is imperative to think of himself or herself as part of a multidisciplinary team. Two-way referrals should occur only through constant communication, understanding of the modalities and with consistent communication with the oncologist. Therefore, appropriate referrals can be achieved. Ultimately, this team approach allows the patient to have greater benefit and allows us to provide the most safe and effective treatment for all patients.

References

1. NIH Consensus Conference. Acupuncture. JAMA 1998; 280:1518–24.
2. Shen J, Wenger N, Glaspy J, et al. Electroacupuncture for control of myeloablative chemotherapy-induced emesis: a randomized controlled trial. JAMA 2000; 284: 2755–61.
3. Wong RK, Jones GW, Sagar SM, Babjak AF, Whelan T. A Phase I-II study in the use of acupuncture-like transcutaneous nerve stimulation in the treatment of radiation-induced xerostomia in head-and-neck cancer patients treated with radical radiotherapy. Int J Radiat Oncol Biol Phys 2003; 57:472–80.
4. Johnstone PA, Peng YP, May BC, Inouye WS, Niemtzow RC. Acupuncture for pilocarpine-resistant xerostomia following radiotherapy for head and neck malignancies. Int J Radiat Oncol Biol Phys 2001; 50:353–7.
5. Johnstone PA, Niemtzow RC, Riffenburgh RH. Acupuncture for xerostomia: clinical update. Cancer 2002; 94:1151–6.
6. Vickers AJ, Straus DJ, Fearon B, Cassileth BR. Acupuncture for postchemotherapy fatigue: a phase II study. J Clin Oncol 2004; 22:1731–5.
7. Wong R, Sagar S. Acupuncture treatment for chemotherapy-induced perepheral neuropathy–a case series, *Acupunct Med.*, 2006 Jun; 24(2):87–91.
8. Alimi D, Rubino C, Pichard-Leandri E, Fermand-Brule S, Dubreuil-Lemaire ML, Hill C. Analgesic effect of auricular acupuncture for cancer pain: a randomized, blinded, controlled trial. J Clin Oncol 2003; 21:4120–6.
9. Wang SM, Gaal D, Maranets I, Caldwell-Andrews A, Kain ZN. Acupressure and preoperative parental anxiety: a pilot study. Anesth Analg 2005; 101:666–9, table of contents.
10. Wang SM, Peloquin C, Kain ZN. The use of auricular acupuncture to reduce preoperative anxiety. Anesth Analg 2001; 93:1178–80, table of contents.
11. He D, Hostmark AT, Veiersted KB, Medbo JI. Effect of intensive acupuncture on pain-related social and psychological variables for women with chronic neck and shoulder pain–an RCT with six month and three year follow up. Acupunct Med 2005; 23:52–61.
12. Spence DW, Kayumov L, Chen A, et al. Acupuncture increases nocturnal melatonin secretion and reduces insomnia and anxiety: a preliminary report. J Neuropsychiatry Clin Neurosci 2004; 16:19–28.

13. Jun EM, Chang S. Kang DH, Kim S. Effects of acupressure on dysmenorrhea and skin temperature changes in college students: a non-randomized controlled trial. Int J Nurs Stud. 2007 Aug; 44(6):973–81
14. Svedberg LE, Nordahl UE, Lundeberg TC. Effects of acupuncture on skin temperature in children with neurological disorders and cold feet: an exploratory study. Complement Ther Med. 2001 Jun; 9(2):89–97.

Chapter 13
Acupuncture for the Side Effects of Cancer Treatments

Sanghoon Lee, Kathleen Menten, and Adrian S. Dobs

Contents

13.1 Introduction	201
13.2 Side Effects of Cancer Treatment	202
13.3 Conclusion and Summary	208
References	208

Abstract Johns Hopkins introduced acupuncture in The Sidney Kimmel Comprehensive Cancer Center in September 2005 to provide an expanded service for our Complementary and Integrative Medicine Center. The current goal of our acupuncture service is predominately to relieve the side effects of cancer treatment. In this chapter, we briefly review current biomedical treatments and any available data on the role of acupuncture for common side effects of cancer therapy, that is, oral mucositis, peripheral neuropathy, nausea/vomiting, and fatigue. The need for integrative cancer care requires good clinical trials to evaluate the possible clinical benefits of acupuncture and to investigate its underlying mechanism.

Keywords: Acupuncture · side effects · cancer treatments · oral mucositis · peripheral neuropathy · nausea · vomiting · fatigue.

13.1 Introduction

Johns Hopkins introduced acupuncture as part of the Complementary and Integrative Medicine service in The Sidney Kimmel Comprehensive Cancer Center in September 2005. The treatment objective of acupuncture in our clinic at Johns

---

A. Dobs
Professor of Medicine and Oncology, Division of Endocrinology & Metabolism, Johns Hopkins University, 1830 East Monument Street, Suite 328, Baltimore, MD 21287
e-mail: adobs@jhmi.edu

L. Cohen, M. Markman (eds.), *Integrative Oncology: Incorporating Complementary Medicine into Conventional Cancer Care*, © 2008 Humana Press, Totowa, NJ

Hopkins is mainly to relieve the side effects of cancer treatment, working as a complement to the conventional treatments given here. The distribution of previous and ongoing cancer treatments for our population of acupuncture clinic patients was chemotherapy (47%), radiation (9%), both (38%), and surgery (6%).

Although current cancer therapies have contributed to increased survival rates in many cancers, they also cause many painful and intractable side effects, which seriously affect the quality of life in cancer patients [1–3]. Therefore, the current goal of acupuncture for cancer patients is to improve the quality of life through a holistic approach which seeks to solve functional problems rather than eradicate a malignant tumor itself [4,5]. This approach can also help patients endure the difficult times during the cancer treatment.

In this chapter, we briefly review major cancer treatment side effects and previous acupuncture studies and introduce possible acupuncture prescriptions. These prescriptions suggested for further study are based on Korean Saam Acupuncture or clinical experience. Modifications should be considered according to patient condition and response. We hope this chapter stimulates cooperation among the Integrative Medicine Services of the major oncology centers.

13.2 Side Effects of Cancer Treatment

13.2.1 Oral Mucositis

13.2.1.1 Clinical Presentation and Standard Option

Oral mucositis is an injury of the oral mucosa [6], which can cause erythema, ulceration, and even tissue necrosis [7]. Specifically, this symptom occurs in 89–100% of patients receiving radiation therapy for head and neck cancers [8], 75% of patients receiving stem cell transplantation [9], and 31% of patients receiving chemotherapy for solid tumors [10]. In a study, 67.4% of myeloablative chemotherapy patients had either grade III ("cannot eat") or grade IV mucositis ("requiring parenteral support or opiate analgesics") [11].

This oral toxicity occurs by DNA and non-DNA damage initiated by radiation or chemotherapy [12]. The mechanism of injury is mediated through reactive oxygen species and proinflammatory cytokines [12]. Keratinocyte growth factor (palifermin) was reported to reduce the incidence and severity of oral mucositis following autologous stem cell transplant with mild adverse events including rash, erythema, edema, and pruritis [13–15]. For patients with non-hematologic malignancy, however, more efficacy and safety evidence should be established due to its potential for unexpected adverse events [16,17]. The conventional interventions (e.g. oral wash, mucosal protectants) are mainly supportive [18], and the mainstay for current mucositis pain relief is the administration of morphine [19, 20]. However, opioids can cause tolerance and physical dependence [19] and other potential side effects such as bradypnoea, hypoxia, nausea and vomiting, sedation, pruritus, and urinary retention [21].

13.2.1.2 Overview of Acupuncture Studies

No acupuncture trial for cancer-related mucositis was published in major databases such as PubMed. If acupuncture can relieve inflammatory pain, its effect may be related with substance P, β-endorphin, and the balance between proinflammatory and anti-inflammatory cytokines such as TNF-α and IL-10 [22].

13.2.1.3 Acupuncture for Mucositis Pain Control - Pilot Study

Mucositis is not only extremely painful, but also devastates quality of life because of increasing risks of infection, and malnutrition. This often leads to discontinuing or delaying chemotherapy. Since there is a need to seek alternatives or adjuvant therapies for mucositis pain control, we are presently planning acupuncture research for mucositis patients. Acupuncture is a possible therapy because it has been shown to be effective for various pain conditions and other cancer treatment side effects such as nausea and vomiting.

The overall goal of our clinical study is to investigate the feasibility, effectiveness, and safety of acupuncture in treating mucositis and relieving its pain. We propose a randomized controlled trial in which mucositis patients will undergo acupuncture vs. sham procedure.

Intervention of the acupuncture procedure is as follows:

Intervention

Acupuncture Group: Real Acupuncture

Participants will receive the acupuncture therapy three times per week on alternating days for a total of 2 weeks (total of six treatments). The main prescriptions will be acupuncture points tonifying the Spleen Meridian and the Small Intestine Meridian on the basis of the Saam Acupuncture theory [23, 24] often known as "four needle technique," although other modified acupuncture prescriptions may be applicable according to the patient's response in this pilot study.

In Oriental Medicine, the Spleen has the functions of promoting fluid metabolism, transporting nutrients, and controlling blood [25]. The mouth belongs to the Spleen system according to Five Element Theory [26]. The Small intestine is related with mucositis symptoms, including oral ulcer and tongue problems because the tongue belongs to the Heart system in Oriental Medicine and the Heart is coupled with the Small intestine in the Five Element Theory [26]. Tonifying the Small intestine prescription is often applied to various ulcerative or inflammatory conditions due to its Taiyang meridian characteristics of cooling excessive heat [23, 24].

SP02 (+), HT08 (+), SP01 (–), LR01 (–); Tonifying Spleen Meridian
SI03 (+), GB44 (+), SI02 (–), BL66 (–); Tonifying Small Intestine Meridian

Note: Manual needling technique in this chapter

- (+): Tonification: needle insertion along the meridian flow; Respiration technique: needle insertion in exhalation, removal in inhalation
- (–): Sedation: needle insertion against the meridian flow; Respiration technique: needle insertion in inhalation, removal in exhalation
- Other needling techniques for tonification or sedation can be combined, if necessary.

Control Group: Sham Acupuncture

Eight sham needles (Park Sham Device, AcuPrime, Exeter, UK) will be applied on non-acupuncture points on the arms and legs. The sham needle has a telescopic needle body with a blunt tip, and this sham device gives the impression of insertion and some pricking sensation without penetrating the skin (Fig. 13.1) [27]. Each needle will be attached on non-acupuncture points between classical meridians for 20 min. Except for the penetration of skin, all other procedures will be the same as the Acupuncture group.

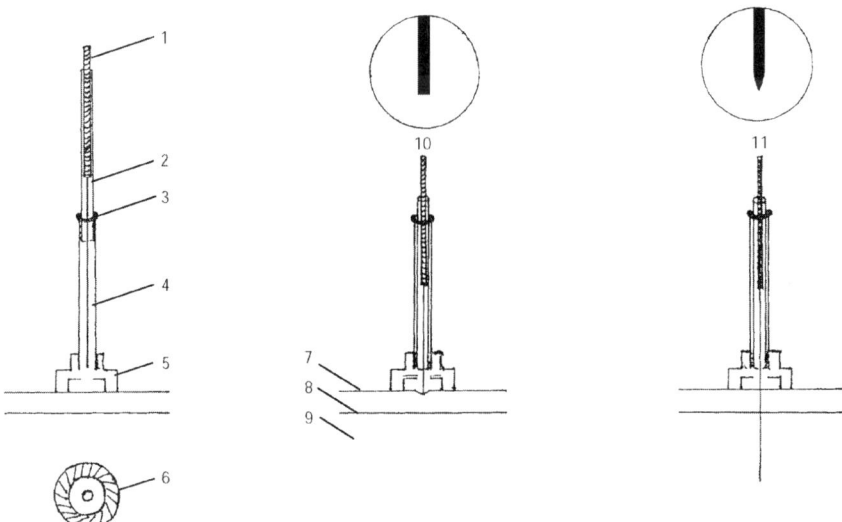

Fig. 13.1 Park Sham Device [27] (by courtesy of JB Park). 1. Needle handle, 2. Guide tube, 3. Guide o-ring, 4. Park tube, 5. Flange, 6. Double-sided tape, 7. Skin, 8. Dermis, 9. Muscle, 10. Dull tip of sham needle, 11. Sharp tip of real needle.

13.2.2 Peripheral Neuropathy

13.2.2.1 Clinical Presentation and Standard Option

Cancer itself can cause peripheral neuropathy by compression or infiltration of nerve tissue; however, neuropathies in cancer patients are more commonly caused by surgery, radiation, and chemotherapy [28]. Surgery or radiotherapy can cause neuropathy in the affected area [29], and various neuro-toxic chemotherapies can damage the peripheral nervous system, including the cell body, axon, and myelin sheath [30]. Sensory or motor dysfunction leads to diverse symptoms from mild weakness, numbness, tingling, burning sensation to uncontrollable pain, and ataxia [29, 31]. Although the neuropathic symptoms are generally not fatal and can be improved after finishing chemotherapy, they often progress and seriously affect patients' quality of life and interfere with cancer treatments [32]. Some of our patients also have indicated that neuropathy has been the worst part of their entire treatment experience.

Current management for peripheral neuropathy is using opioid and adjuvant analgesics including anticonvulsant and antidepressant medications [28, 32]. A recent review reports that glutamine, glutathione, vitamin E, acetyl-L-carnitine, calcium, and magnesium infusions might be helpful for chemotherapy-induced peripheral neuropathy [30]; however, further evidence is required and non-pharmacologic approaches such as exercise and massage can be also considered [33].

13.2.2.2 Overview of Acupuncture Studies

A pilot case study on acupuncture for chemotherapy-induced neuropathy reported that five patients showed an encouraging response after a series of acupuncture treatments [34]. The points used were CV6, ST36, LI11, Ba Feng, and Ba Xie, and, if necessary, tips of affected fingers or toes were needled additionally. One well-designed randomized controlled trial for cancer pain included peripheral or central neuropathic pain patients who were still in a significant amount of pain, despite being treated with opiod analgesics [35]. The authors concluded that auricular acupuncture decreased pain intensity by 36% at 2 months from baseline while there was only a 2% change for patients receiving placebo. The design of this study included an individualized selection of auricular acupuncture points based on the presence of an electrodermal signal on the ear for point detection.

Acupuncture research for peripheral neuropathy in other disease conditions has showed improvement in patients with diabetic neuropathy [36] and HIV [37]. Conversely, another study reported that neither acupuncture nor amitriptyline was more effective than placebo in HIV-related peripheral neuropathic pain [38].

13.2.2.3 Clinical Application

Our acupuncturist here at Johns Hopkins has been using a modified version of Alimi's auricular approach [35] in the treatment of cancer patients with a significant amount of neuropathy, despite the use of opiod analgesics and off label drugs like lyrica and cymbalta, or neurontin and amytriptyline. We use an electro-acupuncture device to locate points on the ear that are responsive to an electrodermal signal. On one ear, acupuncture needles are used; on the other, the electo-acpuncture device is used to both locate and treat the auricular acupuncture points. Additional body acupuncture points are individually selected based on the condition of the patient. Our results have been impressive enough to get the attention of our attending physicians, who are now referring patients for this treatment. (Previously, patients had to be aware of, and ask for a referral for acupuncture.)

13.2.2.4 Recommendation for Acupuncture in the Treatment of Peripheral Neuropathy

Peripheral neuropathy manifests in many different ways. Saam Acupuncture recommends the treatment of neuropathy-like symptoms as below [23].

- Moving or spreading pain
  GB44 (+), LI01 (+), GB38 (−), SI05 (−)
- Fixed or spot pain, aggravated with coldness
  LI05 (+), SI05 (+), LI02 (−), BL66 (−)
- Burning or erythematous pain
  SI03 (+), GB41 (+), SI02 (−), BL66 (−)
- Skin pain with numbness or itching
  LU09 (+), SP03 (+), LU10 (−), HT08 (−)

13.2.3 Nausea/Vomiting

13.2.3.1 Clinical Presentation and Standard Treatment Options

Nausea and vomiting are very common side effects of chemotherapy for cancer. Acute nausea and vomiting occurs within the first 24 hour after chemotherapy; delayed nausea and vomiting occurs 24 hours to several days after start of chemotherapy; and anticipatory nausea and vomiting are triggered by taste, odor, sight, thoughts, or anxiety secondary to a history of poor response to antiemetic agents [39].

The release of serotonin seems to play a role in initiating the vomiting reflex, and the administration of serotonin receptor antagonists is effective to control nausea and vomiting [40, 41]. Current standard option for nausea and vomiting for cancer patients is the combination of a 5-hydroxytryptamine-3 serotonin receptor antagonist, dexamethasone, and aprepitant according to emetic risk level [42].

However, many poor responders in the delayed phase [43] and high antiemetic costs [44] often require other possible alternatives.

13.2.3.2 Overview of Acupuncture Studies for Nausea and Vomiting

Nausea and vomiting have been a well-known indication of acupuncture for cancer patients. Many reports on the efficacy of acupuncture for these symptoms were published, including Dundee et al.'s several reports [45–49] and the National Institute of Health Consensus Statement on Acupuncture [50].

A meta-analysis study reported that pericardium point 6 (PC6, *Neiguan*) is the most commonly used acupuncture point and that various modalities such as manual acupuncture, electroacupuncture, and acupressure can be applied [51]. This review article concluded that electroacupuncture is beneficial for chemotherapy-induced acute vomiting and acupressure seems to diminish acute nausea severity.

Recently, Streitberger et al. [52] summarized possible mechanisms of acupuncture effects on nausea and vomiting; neurotransmitters, smooth muscle of the gut, somatovisceral reflex, sensory input inhibition, somatosympathetic reflex, vagal modulation, and cerebellar vestibular activities. However, the clear mechanism is unknown at the moment.

13.2.3.3 Recommendation for Acupuncture Treatment for Nausea and Vomiting

As above, nausea and vomiting can be controlled with modern antiemetic drugs [42], and stimulating PC6 is an effective non-pharmacological treatment [52]. However, for poor responders to conventional therapies, the following acupuncture prescription for tonifying Spleen Meridian can be applied according to Saam Acupuncture [23].

SP02 (+), HT08 (+), SP01 (−), LR01 (−)

13.2.4 Fatigue

13.2.4.1 Clinical Presentation and Standard Treatment Options

As much as 78% of cancer patients experienced fatigue, and 32% of these patients experienced fatigue daily, which significantly affected their daily routines [53]. The reasons for cancer-related fatigue are complicated: cancer itself, cytotoxic treatment, systemic disorders (anemia, malnutrition, or renal insufficiency, etc.), sleep disturbance, lack of exercise, pain, and emotional distress [54]. After identifying and treating the above factors, remaining interventions to relieve fatigue are mainly for symptom management and emotional support. Exercise, energy conservation and activity, education, relaxation, and massage can be recommended to overcome fatigue [55].

13.2.4.2 Overview of Acupuncture Studies

In a phase II study, post-chemotherapy fatigue patients showed 31.1% improvement on the Brief Fatigue Inventory from baseline to follow-up after receiving acupuncture treatment twice weekly for 4 weeks or once weekly for 6 weeks [56]. There are several favorable reports on the effect of electroacupuncture for chronic fatigue syndrome: electroacupuncture with auricular-plaster therapy [57], electroacupuncture on back-shu points [58], and electroacupuncture on LI 11 and ST 36 [59].

13.2.4.3 Recommendation of Acupuncture for Fatigue

From the view of Oriental Medicine, radiation or chemotherapy damages the Yin fluids and the visceral energy (or Qi), especially Spleen Qi, which is related with movement and circulation of QI and blood in our body [60]. Spleen energy's malfunction may lead to tiredness and heavy feeling and indigestion [25,26]. Therefore, tonifying Spleen energy could help relieve fatigue, and other alternative prescriptions can be applied according to Saam Acupuncture [23, 24].

SP02 (+), HT08 (+), SP01 (−), LR01 (−); Tonifying Spleen Meridian
SP03 (+), LU09 (+), TE06 (−), KI02 (−); alternative option for phyisical fatigue
LU08 (+), SP03 (+), HT 08 (+), CV 06 (−), BL (15) (−); alternative option for mental fatigue

13.3 Conclusion and Summary

Side effects of cancer treatments have a detrimental impact on quality of life for patients. Acupuncture has been applied for various conditions including pain control. Its research in this area is ripe for good clinical trials to evaluate the possible benefits of acupuncture.

Acknowledgments This manuscript has been supported in part by grant number AT00437 from the National Center for Complementary & Alternative Medicine of the National Institutes of Health; Adrian S. Dobs, MD MHS, Principal Investigator; by a grant from the Kimmel Foundation; and by Kyung Hee University, Seoul, Korea.

References

1. Sun CC, Ramirez PT, Bodurka DC. Quality of life for patients with epithelial ovarian cancer. *Nat Clin Pract Oncol* Jan 2007;4(1):18–29.
2. Vistad I, Fossa SD, Dahl AA. A critical review of patient-rated quality of life studies of long-term survivors of cervical cancer. *Gynecol Oncol* Sep 2006;102(3):563–572.
3. Scalliet PG, Remouchamps V, Curran D, et al. Retrospective analysis of results of p(65)+Be neutron therapy for treatment of prostate adenocarcinoma at the cyclotron of Louvain-la-Leuve. Part II: Side effects and their influence on quality of life measured with QLQ-C30 of EORTC. *Int J Radiat Oncol Biol Phys* Apr 1 2004;58(5):1549–1561.
4. Lu W. Acupuncture for side effects of chemoradiation therapy in cancer patients. *Semin Oncol Nurs* Aug 2005;21(3):190–195.

5. Cohen AJ, Menter A, Hale L. Acupuncture: role in comprehensive cancer care–a primer for the oncologist and review of the literature. *Integr Cancer Ther* Jun 2005;4(2): 131–143.
6. Stokman MA, Spijkervet FK, Boezen HM, Schouten JP, Roodenburg JL, de Vries EG. Preventive intervention possibilities in radiotherapy- and chemotherapy-induced oral mucositis: results of meta-analyses. *J Dent Res* Aug 2006;85(8):690–700.
7. National Cancer Institute Common Toxicity Criteria available. http://ctep.cancer.gov/forms/CTCAEv3.pdf. Accessed September 12, 2006.
8. Trotti A, Bellm LA, Epstein JB, et al. Mucositis incidence, severity and associated outcomes in patients with head and neck cancer receiving radiotherapy with or without chemotherapy: a systematic literature review. *Radiother Oncol* Mar 2003;66(3):253–262.
9. Stiff P. Mucositis associated with stem cell transplantation: current status and innovative approaches to management. *Bone Marrow Transplant* May 2001;27 Suppl 2: S3–S11.
10. Raber-Durlacher JE, Weijl NI, Abu Saris M, de Koning B, Zwinderman AH, Osanto S. Oral mucositis in patients treated with chemotherapy for solid tumors: a retrospective analysis of 150 cases. *Support Care Cancer* Sep 2000;8(5):366–371.
11. Wardley AM, Jayson GC, Swindell R, et al. Prospective evaluation of oral mucositis in patients receiving myeloablative conditioning regimens and haemopoietic progenitor rescue. *Br J Haematol* Aug 2000;110(2):292–299.
12. Sonis ST. The pathobiology of mucositis. *Nat Rev Cancer* Apr 2004;4(4):277–284.
13. Spielberger R, Stiff P, Bensinger W, et al. Palifermin for oral mucositis after intensive therapy for hematologic cancers. *N Engl J Med* Dec 16 2004;351(25):2590–2598.
14. Beaven AW, Shea TC. Palifermin: a keratinocyte growth factor that reduces oral mucositis after stem cell transplant for haematological malignancies. *Expert Opin Pharmacother* Nov 2006;7(16):2287–2299.
15. Radtke ML, Kolesar JM. Palifermin (Kepivance) for the treatment of oral mucositis in patients with hematologic malignancies requiring hematopoietic stem cell support. *J Oncol Pharm Pract* Sep 2005;11(3):121–125.
16. Safety&Tolerability. http://www.kepivance.com/kepivance/safety_tolerability.jsp. Accessed August 29, 2006.
17. McDonnell AM, Lenz KL. Palifermin: role in the prevention of chemotherapy- and radiation-induced mucositis. *Ann Pharmacother* Jan 2007;41(1):86–94.
18. Worthington HV, Clarkson JE, Eden OB. Interventions for treating oral mucositis for patients with cancer receiving treatment. *Cochrane Database Syst Rev* 2002(1):CD001973.
19. Coda BA, O'Sullivan B, Donaldson G, Bohl S, Chapman CR, Shen DD. Comparative efficacy of patient-controlled administration of morphine, hydromorphone, or sufentanil for the treatment of oral mucositis pain following bone marrow transplantation. *Pain* Sep 1997;72(3): 333–346.
20. Cerchietti LC, Navigante AH, Bonomi MR, et al. Effect of topical morphine for mucositis-associated pain following concomitant chemoradiotherapy for head and neck carcinoma. *Cancer* Nov 15 2002;95(10):2230–2236.
21. Walder B, Schafer M, Henzi I, Tramer MR. Efficacy and safety of patient-controlled opioid analgesia for acute postoperative pain. A quantitative systematic review. *Acta Anaesthesiol Scand* Aug 2001;45(7):795–804.
22. Zijlstra FJ, van den Berg-de Lange I, Huygen FJ, Klein J. Anti-inflammatory actions of acupuncture. *Mediators Inflamm* Apr 2003;12(2):59–69.
23. Kim DH. *Saam Doin Chimbeop*. 4 ed. Pusan: Sogang Press; 2004.
24. Kim KJ. *Woloh Saam Ohaeng Chimbeop*. 2 ed. Seoul: Iljungsa; 2005.
25. Zhang E. *Basic Theory of Traditional Chinese Medicine*. Shanghai: Publishing House of Shanghai College of Traditional Chinese Medicine; 1989.
26. Maciocia G. *The Foundations of Chinese Medicine*. New York: Churchill Livingstone; 1989.
27. Park J, White A, Stevinson C, Ernst E, James M. Validating a new non-penetrating sham acupuncture device: two randomised controlled trials. *Acupunct Med* Dec 2002;20(4): 168–174.

28. Forman A. Peripheral neuropathy in cancer patients: clinical types, etiology, and presentation. Part 2. *Oncology (Williston Park).* Feb 1990;4(2):85–89.
29. Polomano RC, Farrar JT. Pain and neuropathy in cancer survivors. *Cancer Nurs* Mar–Apr 2006;29(2 Suppl):39–47.
30. Stillman M, Cata JP. Management of chemotherapy-induced peripheral neuropathy. *Curr Pain Headache Rep* Aug 2006;10(4):279–287.
31. Forman A. Peripheral neuropathy in cancer patients: incidence, features, and pathophysiology. *Oncology (Williston Park).* Jan 1990;4(1):57–62 concl.
32. Forman AD. Peripheral neuropathy and cancer. *Curr Oncol Rep* Jan 2004;6(1):20–25.
33. Armstrong T, Almadrones L, Gilbert MR. Chemotherapy-induced peripheral neuropathy. *Oncol Nurs Forum* Mar 2005;32(2):305–311.
34. Wong R, Sagar S. Acupuncture treatment for chemotherapy-induced peripheral neuropathy–a case series. *Acupunct Med* Jun 2006;24(2):87–91.
35. Alimi D, Rubino C, Pichard-Leandri E, Fermand-Brule S, Dubreuil-Lemaire ML, Hill C. Analgesic effect of auricular acupuncture for cancer pain: a randomized, blinded, controlled trial. *J Clin Oncol* Nov 15 2003;21(22):4120–4126.
36. Abuaisha BB, Costanzi JB, Boulton AJ. Acupuncture for the treatment of chronic painful peripheral diabetic neuropathy: a long-term study. *Diabetes Res Clin Pract* Feb 1998;39(2):115–121.
37. Phillips KD, Skelton WD, Hand GA. Effect of acupuncture administered in a group setting on pain and subjective peripheral neuropathy in persons with human immunodeficiency virus disease. *J Altern Complement Med* Jun 2004;10(3):449–455.
38. Shlay JC, Chaloner K, Max MB, et al. Acupuncture and amitriptyline for pain due to HIV-related peripheral neuropathy: a randomized controlled trial. Terry Beirn Community Programs for Clinical Research on AIDS. *JAMA* Nov 11 1998;280(18):1590–1595.
39. Jordan K, Kasper C, Schmoll HJ. Chemotherapy-induced nausea and vomiting: current and new standards in the antiemetic prophylaxis and treatment. *Eur J Cancer* Jan 2005;41(2):199–205.
40. Hesketh PJ. Comparative review of 5-HT3 receptor antagonists in the treatment of acute chemotherapy-induced nausea and vomiting. *Cancer Invest* 2000;18(2):163–173.
41. Guerra MC. Acupuncture for refractory cases of chemotherapy-induced nausea and vomiting. *Med Acupunct* 2004;16(1):40–42.
42. Kris MG, Hesketh PJ, Somerfield MR, et al. American Society of Clinical Oncology Guideline for Antiemetics in Oncology: Update 2006. *J Clin Oncol* Jun 20 2006;24(18):2932–2947.
43. Grunberg SM, Deuson RR, Mavros P, et al. Incidence of chemotherapy-induced nausea and emesis after modern antiemetics. *Cancer* May 15 2004;100(10):2261–2268.
44. Ihbe-Heffinger A, Ehlken B, Bernard R, et al. The impact of delayed chemotherapy-induced nausea and vomiting on patients, health resource utilization and costs in German cancer centers. *Ann Oncol* Mar 2004;15(3):526–536.
45. Dundee JW, Ghaly RG, Fitzpatrick KT, Lynch GA, Abram WP. Acupuncture to prevent cisplatin-associated vomiting. *Lancet* May 9 1987;1(8541):1083.
46. Dundee JW, Ghaly RG, Fitzpatrick KT, Abram WP, Lynch GA. Acupuncture prophylaxis of cancer chemotherapy-induced sickness. *J R Soc Med* May 1989;82(5):268–271.
47. Dundee JW, McMillan CM. Clinical uses of P6 acupuncture antiemesis. *Acupunct Electrother Res* 1990;15(3–4):211–215.
48. Dundee JW, Yang J. Prolongation of the antiemetic action of P6 acupuncture by acupressure in patients having cancer chemotherapy. *J R Soc Med* Jun 1990;83(6):360–362.
49. Dundee JW, Yang J, McMillan C. Non-invasive stimulation of the P6 (Neiguan) antiemetic acupuncture point in cancer chemotherapy. *J R Soc Med* Apr 1991;84(4):210–212.
50. NIH Consensus Conference. Acupuncture. *JAMA* Nov 4 1998;280(17):1518–1524.
51. Ezzo JM, Richardson MA, Vickers A, et al. Acupuncture-point stimulation for chemotherapy-induced nausea or vomiting. *Cochrane Database Syst Rev* 2006(2):CD002285.
52. Streitberger K, Ezzo J, Schneider A. Acupuncture for nausea and vomiting: an update of clinical and experimental studies. *Auton Neurosci* Oct 30 2006;129(1–2):107–117.

53. Vogelzang NJ, Breitbart W, Cella D, et al. Patient, caregiver, and oncologist perceptions of cancer-related fatigue: results of a tripart assessment survey. The Fatigue Coalition. *Semin Hematol* Jul 1997;34(3 Suppl 2):4–12.
54. Madden J, Newton S. Why am I so tired all the time? Understanding cancer-related fatigue. *Clin J Oncol Nurs* Oct 2006;10(5):659–661.
55. Mitchell SA, Berger AM. Cancer-related fatigue: the evidence base for assessment and management. *Cancer J* Sep–Oct 2006;12(5):374–387.
56. Vickers AJ, Straus DJ, Fearon B, Cassileth BR. Acupuncture for postchemotherapy fatigue: a phase II study. *J Clin Oncol* May 1 2004;22(9):1731–1735.
57. Yuemei L, Hongping L, Shulan F, Dongfang G. The therapeutic effects of electrical acupuncture and auricular-plaster in 32 cases of chronic fatigue syndrome. *J Tradit Chin Med* Sep 2006;26(3):163–164.
58. Wang Q, Xiong JX. Clinical observation on effect of electro-acupuncture on back-shu points in treating chronic fatigue syndrome. *Zhongguo Zhong Xi Yi Jie He Za Zhi* Sep 2005;25(9): 834–836.
59. Mears T. Acupuncture in the treatment of post viral fatigue syndrome–a case report. *Acupunct Med* Sep 2005;23(3):141–145.
60. Li P, Cheng Z, Du X. *Management of Cancer with Chinese Medicine*. Mao S, Bao L, trans. Albans: Donica Publishing Ltd; 2003:189–208.

Index

AboutHerbs Web site (www.mskcc.org/aboutherbs), 77–78
Acupuncture, 74–75
　in cancer center, 191–198
　for cancer pain, 189
　cancer treatments side effects and, 199
　　fatigue, 205–206
　　nausea/vomiting, 204–205
　　oral mucositis, 200–202
　　peripheral neuropathy, 203–204
　for chemotherapy-related neuropathy, 189
　contraindications and precautions in, 190–191
　credentialing policy, at DFCI, 85–87
　at DFCI, 84–85, 182–183
　　documentation, 184
　　standardized approach for, 185
　hot flash therapy, 127
　insomnia and anxiety, 190
　at Johns Hopkins CIM Service, 110
　meridian theory, 17
　nausea/vomiting, 188
　oncology, 185–187
　for post-chemotherapy-related fatigue, 189
　for radiotherapy-induced xerostomia, 188
Advanced cancer, treatments, 130–131
Advanced solid tumors, huanglian for, 163–166
American Cancer Society, 170
Amygdalin (laetrile), 130
Anderson Network Conference, 50–51
Anorexia and cachexia, 128–130
Anticoagulants, 191

Baicalein, 173
Bendheim Integrative Medicine Center, 70, 72, 75
Benzodiazepines, 162

Black cohosh, as herb for hot flashes, 127
Blastocystis hominis, 163
Botanicals, 162. *See also* Specific types
Breast cancer, 125, 150
　maitake in, 170–172

CAM therapies, 15
　acupuncture. *See* Acupuncture
　broader ethical analysis, 28–30
　at DFCI, 80–81, 83, 98–100
　liability risks, management of, 26–27
　major applicable legal rules, 16
　　licensure and credentialing, 17–18
　　malpractice, 19
　　professional discipline, third-party reimbursement, and healthcare fraud, 19–20
　　scope of practice, 18–19
　malpractice issues. *See* Malpractice issues, CAM therapies and
　massage therapy. *See* Massage therapy, for cancer patients
　meditation, 144–147, 152
　state medical board guidelines for, 27–28
Cancer pain, acupuncture for, 189
Cancer Patient Education Network (CPEN), 98
Capsaicin, 128
Center for Holistic Pediatric Education and Research (CHPER), 95
Chemotherapy, 42, 74
　acupuncture and, 188–189
Chinese herbal medicine (CHM), 183
Chronic hepatitis C, SST for, 172–175
Chronic neuropathic pain, 128
Cognitive behavioral therapy, 22. *See also* CAM therapies
Communication, in cancer care, 35–36
　between physicians and CIM practitioners, 39–43

Communication, in cancer care *(cont.)*
  patient's perspective, 37–38
  physician's perspective, 38
Complementary and alternative medicine (CAM), 3–6, 12, 59–60, 106, 140
  multi-institutional courses for, 61
  potential "harms" associated with, 10–11
  therapies. *See* CAM therapies
Complementary and integrative medicine (CIM) therapies, in cancer care, 34
  approaching strategy for use of, 41–43
  communication and, 35–36
    between physicians and CIM practitioners, 39–43
    patient's perspective, 37–38
    physician's perspective, 38
  integrative medicine program and, 51–52, 54
  Johns Hopkins Medical Institutions and. *See* Johns Hopkins Complementary and Integrative Medicine Service
Complementary/Integrative Medicine Education Resources (CIMER) Web site, 55, 57–59, 63
  Patient/provider communication and, 59–60
Coptis chinesis. See Huanglian, for patients with advanced solid tumors
Corticosteroids, 128
Creatine, 129–130
Cytochrome P450 3A4, 162

Dana-Farber Cancer Institute (DFCI), Zakim Center for Integrative Oncology, 79
  acupuncture at, 84–85, 182–183
    documentation, 184
    standardized approach for, 185
  collaborations, 93–94
  development of, 80–81
  financials, 96–98
  growth of, 94–96
  integrative education program creation, 98–102
  integrative therapies, documentation and scheduling of, 91–93
  mission statement, 81–83
  policies and procedures, 83–91
Dehydroepiandrosterone (DHEA), hot flash remedy, 125, 127
Dexamethasone, 162
Docetaxel with Jin Fu Kang, for patients with NSCLC, 166–170

Eicosapentaenoic acid (EPA), 129
Electroacupuncture, 85, 188, 193. *See also* Acupuncture
Electronic medical record (EMR), 82, 91

Fatigue, as cancer treatment side effect, 205–206
  acupuncture for, 189
Food and Drug Administration (FDA), 12, 59, 163, 192

Ginseng, 173
Glycyrrhizin, 173
Graft *versus* host (GVH) reaction, 167
Green tea, treatment for cancer, 130
Grifola frondosa. See Maitake, in breast cancer

Heliobacter pylori, 163
Hepatitis C virus (HCV), 172
Hepatocellular carcinoma (HCC), 173
Herbal supplements, for cancer patient, 162–163
High performance liquid chromatography (HPLC), 164–165, 169
Huanglian, for patients with advanced solid tumors, 163–166
Hydrazine sulfate, 128–129
Hypnotherapy, 15

Icariin, 169
"Important Conversations: Complementary Therapies and Cancer", 60
Insomnia and anxiety, acupuncture for, 190
Integrative Medicine Consultation, 111
Integrative Medicine Program, at University of Texas M. D. Anderson Cancer Center, 49
  clinical delivery
    beginnings, 50–51
    credentialing process, programs, and services, 53–55
    funding, 56
    mission and scope, development, 51–53
    operational areas, 56–57
    registration and screening, 55
    screening and processing program proposals, 53
  education
    internal collaborations, 62
    program evaluation and assessment, 62–63
    programs, 57–61
    marketing, 63–64
    research, 64

Index

Integrative Medicine Service, at Memorial Sloan-Kettering Cancer Center (MSKCC), 67
  clinical services, 70–72
  emergence of, 68–69
  role of, 69–70
  therapies and related research
    AboutHerbs Web site (www.mskcc.org/aboutherbs), 77–78
    acupuncture, 74–75
    education and training, 77
    immune-modulating botanicals research, 76–77
    mind-body therapies, 75
    movement/fitness program, 75–76
    music therapy, 73
    nutrition, 76
    touch therapy, 72–73
  "IntegrativeOncology Fellowship Training program", 77
Interferon (IFN) based therapy, 172–173
Interleukin (IL)10-secreting cells, 148
Internet protocol TV (IPTV) system, 60

Jin Fu Kang with docetaxel, for patients with NSCLC, 166–170
Johns Hopkins Complementary and Integrative Medicine Service, 105
  acupuncture, 110
  case study, 116–117
  challenges faced by, 118
  CIM service administration, 111–113
  clinical service initial stage development process, 106–108
  consultation services, 111
  education programs, 115
  financial aspects, 113–115
  massage therapy, 110–111
  mind-body class, 111
  practical aspects in planning of, 108–110

Karnofsky Performance Status (KPS) Scale, 195
Kimmel Foundation, 107

LACE Program (Longitudinal Ambulatory Care Experience), 61
Leonard P. Zakim Center at DFCI, for integrative oncology, 79
  acupuncture at, 84–85, 182–183
    documentation, 184
    standardized approach for, 185
  collaborations, 93–94
  development of, 80–81
  financials, 96–98
  growth of, 94–96
  integrative education program creation, 98–102
  integrative therapies, documentation and scheduling of, 91–93
  mission statement, 81–83
  policies and procedures, 83–91
Lycopene, for androgen-independent prostate cancer, 131

M. D. Anderson Cancer Center, Integrative Medicine Program, 49
  clinical delivery
    beginnings, 50–51
    credentialing process, programs, and services, 53–55
    funding, 56
    mission and scope, development, 51–53
    operational areas, 56–57
    registration and screening, 55
    screening and processing program proposals, 53
  education
    internal collaborations, 62
    program evaluation and assessment, 62–63
    programs, 57–61
  marketing, 63–64
  research, 64
M.D. Anderson Community Clinical Oncology Program (CCOP), 152
Maitake, in breast cancer, 170–172
Malpractice issues, CAM therapies and, 20
  cancer medicine
    failure to treat in, 21–24
    informed consent in, 24–25
    misdiagnosis in, 21
    referral liability in, 25–26
Massage therapy, for cancer patients, 61
  at Johns Hopkins CIM Service, 110–111
  policy, at DFCI, 87–88
Mayo Clinic, integrative oncology, 123
  research in, 124
    advanced cancer, treatment for, 130–131
    anorexia/cachexia, 128–130
    education, 131–132
    hot flashes, 125–127
    pain, 128
    patient care, 133–134
Meditation, 144–147, 152
Megestrol acetate (MA), 128

Memorial Sloan-Kettering Cancer Center (MSKCC) Integrative Medicine Service, 67
  clinical services, 70–72
  emergence of, 68–69
  role of, 69–70
  therapies and related research
    AboutHerbs Web site (www.mskcc.org/aboutherbs), 77–78
    acupuncture, 74–75
    education and training, 77
    immune-modulating botanicals research, 76–77
    mind-body therapies, 75
    movement/fitness program, 75–76
    music therapy, 73
    nutrition, 76
    touch therapy, 72–73
Mind-body techniques, 22, 75, 83, 139. *See also* CAM therapies
  connection, 141–143
  at Johns Hopkins CIM Service, 111
  limitations, 153–154
  research, at M.D. Anderson
    meditation, 144–147, 152
    Qigong, 147–148, 152–153
    Yoga, 143–144, 148–151
  utilization of, 140–141
Mindfulness-Based Cognitive Therapy (MBCT), 146
Mindfulness-Based Stress Reduction (MBSR), 142, 145–147
Mindfulness relaxation (MR), 152
MKN-74 cells, 164
Movement/Fitness Program, 75–76
Multidisciplinary Care Centers (MCC), at DFCI, 100
Music therapy, 73

N-butyl-N-butanolnitrosoamine, 171
National Breast Cancer Coalition Conference, 116
National Center for Complementary and Alternative Medicine (NCCAM), 3, 5–6, 95, 101, 107
National Certification Commission for Acupuncture and Oriental Medicine (NCCAOM), 109–110, 112
Nausea/vomiting, 204–205
Neutropenia, 190–191
Non-small cell lung cancer (NSCLC), Jin Fu Kang with docetaxel for, 166–170
North Central Cancer Treatment Group (NCCTG), 125, 128, 131

Nu Zhen Zi (*Ligustri lucidum*), 168
Nutritional counseling program, 76

Oncology acupuncture, 185–187
Ondansetron, 162
Oral mucositis, 200–202

Patient-centered care, 34
  patient–physician communication and, 36–37, 40–42
Peripheral neuropathy, 203–204
Physical Medicine and Rehabilitation Services, 54–55
Phytomedicinals. *See* Botanicals
Post-chemotherapy-related fatigue, acupuncture for, 189
Prostate-specific antigen (PSA), 130
Psychosocial support therapy (PST), 148
PubMed., 201

Qigong, 75, 93, 100–101, 147–148, 152–153

Radiotherapy, 42, 144
  induced xerostomia, acupuncture for, 188
Relaxation therapies, 22. *See also* CAM therapies

Shan Zhu Yu (Cornus officinalis), 168
Shark cartilage, for cancer treatment, 131
Shiatsu, massage technique, 72–73
Sho-saiko-to (SST), for chronic hepatitis C, 172–175
Soy phytoestrogens, hot flash remedy, 126–127
Stress Reduction and Relaxation Program (SR-RP), 142

Tai chi, 148
Thrombocytopenia, 191
Touch therapy, 72–73
Transcendental Meditation (TM), 142, 145
Tum-mo, Tibetan meditative practice, 142

Vitamin E, hot flash remedy, 125–126
Vivekananda Yoga Research Foundation, 151

World Health Organization, 112

Xerostomia, radiation-induced, 110, 188
Xiao-Chai Hu-tang, 173

Yin Yang Huo (Epimedium sagittatum), 168–169
Yoga, 143–144, 148–151

Zakim Center. *See* Leonard P. Zakim Center at DFCI, for integrative oncology